NATURAL BEAUTY
SKIN CARE

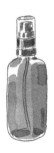

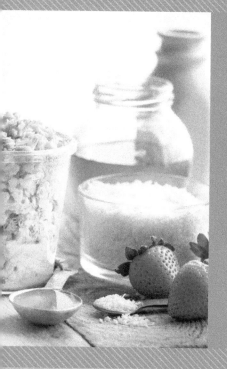

LOVE THE SKIN YOU'RE IN!

Break it off with store-bought beauty products and make your own, the natural way.

- Rejuvenate pores with a detoxing cleanser (page 56)

- Indulge skin with a little sparkling wine (page 85)

- Do the best for your body with a silky goat milk body butter (page 117)

- Don't forget your hair—achieve shiny and soft locks with an Argan oil shampoo (page 128)

There's tons more, for everything from nose to toes!

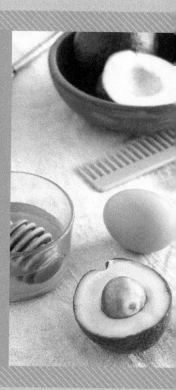

NATURAL BEAUTY
SKIN CARE

110 ORGANIC FORMULAS FOR A RADIANT YOU!

Deborah Burnes

Photography by
Shannon Douglas

ROCKRIDGE
PRESS

For general information on our other products and services or to obtain technical support, please contact our Customer Care Department within the United States at (866) 744–2665, or outside the United States at (510) 253–0500.

Rockridge Press publishes its books in a variety of electronic and print formats. Some content that appears in print may not be available in electronic books, and vice versa.

TRADEMARKS: Rockridge Press and the Rockridge Press logo are trademarks or registered trademarks of Callisto Media Inc. and/or its affiliates, in the United States and other countries, and may not be used without written permission. All other trademarks are the property of their respective owners. Rockridge Press is not associated with any product or vendor mentioned in this book.

Photography © Shannon Douglas
Illustrations © Tom Bingham

ISBN: Print 978-1-62315-664-0
eBook 978-1-62315-665-7

CONTENTS

PREFACE

My desire to educate and empower consumers about cosmetic chemicals and healthy alternatives comes from many sources. I truly love skin—it continues to fascinate and impress me. I love helping people reach their goals, feel good, and be healthy. I have also been blessed with a deep love for many women who have touched me in my life and inspired me to want to help shape our image of beauty, our desire for perfection, and raise awareness about the chemicals in the products we use to achieve this. Beyond education, I feel strongly about using my expertise to offer solutions. This book is dedicated to the many women who have and continue to touch and shape my life.

Women, especially in our society, are preyed upon from the time they can walk down a beauty aisle. With everything from candy-flavored lip balms to the brightly colored packaging on kids' cosmetics (yes, they do make makeup for tots!), companies are seducing future cosmetic devotees. Not only are we bombarded with images in magazines that are unrealistic, we have contests to determine who is the most beautiful . . . starting with babies! And where are the male versions of these contests? Obtaining this image of beauty is sold to us as the ultimate dream from the time we can see and hear and continues throughout our entire lives.

Unfortunately this is a double whammy for women. Who we are and how we feel should not be defined by what is deemed attractive. Young girls should be unaware of their outsides and be able to develop and concentrate on what's inside. On top of the pressure to look a certain way, the products we are being sold to achieve this image are filled with toxic chemicals, harming us and our planet. With both a rise in cancers and studies that show cosmetic chemicals being found in everything from the umbilical cord of unborn babies to breast tumors, we need to take note. We are not only subjecting our daughters to unneeded mental stress but also filling our bodies with a toxic burden. Discussing, changing, and educating on this topic is something I feel strongly about. This is where I can help and enable consumers to make choices—choices they are comfortable with for themselves and their families—as well as offer alternatives to achieve their goals.

Whereas we do not yet understand the complete role cosmetic chemicals have on our health, if we can begin to eliminate toxins from our lives we can reduce the overall chemical burden and stress to our bodies.

The support and encouragement from my friends has been a source of strength. This powerful group of beautiful women aging gracefully, naturally, and comfortably has shown me what beauty really is. Working with celebrities who have to maintain a "look" in an effort to be marketable and get jobs gives me an insight into the conflict and pain that aging brings. Having their careers based upon not only talent but also their appearance visibly makes aging in the public eye a difficult process. Many women in my life still have emotional moments when they look in the mirror (even without the added pressure of Hollywood). Yet without the same pressures, these women can use this as a time to look within, heal, and embrace this new phase of life.

This is not to confuse enjoying self-care with "having" to look a certain way to feel beautiful and chasing unrealistic goals of the images we deem are "perfect," along with the

oodles of products that claim to "enhance," "fix," or even cover "imperfections." Many women undeniably enjoy the art of pampering, dressing up, and wearing makeup. For me I love a night out where I wear makeup, spend way too long picking out an outfit, and have my hair done. I am also comfortable in workout clothes with no makeup and the wrinkles on my face that show the signs of my life. I take care of my skin, enjoy pampering, and refuse to succumb to having to look 20 at 50 or needing to slather chemicals on myself in the name of beauty. To be clear, I am not condemning the age-old art of bathing, pampering, makeup, or any other self-care method that brings you joy. I am offering a peek at some ingredients in most of the products used, discussing how they are harmful, and offering potent and powerful alternatives that will garner the results you are after as well as a reminder of what we all know—that beauty is from within, and we can't find it in a bottle. And to encourage our daughters to feel as comfortable with themselves in sweats and no makeup as they are when they are "done up." If their self-value is not connected with their appearance, we have made strides. And if we can stop the practice of exposing ourselves to toxic chemicals to enhance, fix, or cover, we are on our way.

Here is my gift to all the young women who are looking to love and pamper themselves while staying chemical and toxin free. It is your generation who can make the choices and create the changes for true beauty, and pure products.

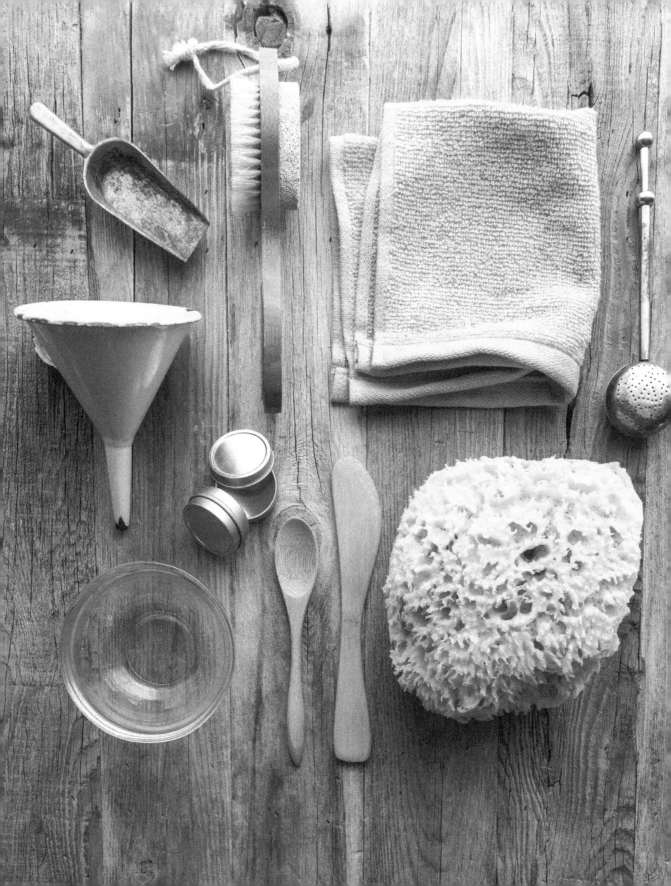

INTRODUCTION

My journey toward healthy skin began early in life. My grandfather was a horticulturist, and I grew up in his garden, learning to identify plants, botanicals, and herbs, which cultivated an excitement for plant life. Over the years I spent several years working as a model for famed artist Salvador Dalí, and clocked some time behind the camera, which gave me a fascination for the transformation that healthy skin, hair, and quality makeup can provide.

Through my work as a model, I realized how much damage the use of heavy makeup and constant hair styling can do. This, plus my passion for plants, led me to study medical herbs and chemistry, and attend cosmetology school. I thought I was just going to understand more of what people were doing to prep me and other models for the camera, but I became obsessed with what I was learning about skin care. I am as crazy about skin now as I was when I first

This book gives me the opportunity to share with you not only fun DIY products you can create at home, but treatments that will transform your skin and help eliminate many of the toxic chemicals from your life.

started school. The marriage of all my loves—chemistry, healing plants, and skin—led me to create my own skin-care products. Soon, friends and family were lining up to use my formulations, and we began to see real results.

In 1999, after searching for truly natural skin-care products in the over-the-counter (OTC) market, a friend and I came up empty-handed. Even in the "natural" skin-care aisle and at health food stores, we found only chemical-laden products. That's when our company *Sum*body was born, long before operating a clean and green company was profitable.

*Sum*body was, and is, about efficacy—our products are nontoxic and effective, and we use only low-waste packaging. We rebranded the term "natural" in skin care as truly free of toxic chemicals, hip, sassy, and good for you. Plus, we aim high—the mass market, not just a small subset. Because education and empowering consumers are as important to me as the products I develop, this book gives me the opportunity to share with you, not only fun DIY products you can create at home, but also treatments that will transform your skin and help eliminate many of the toxic chemicals from your life.

I encourage you to take your DIY enthusiasm to new heights; it is my pleasure to assist in your success. With my years of experience and expertise, I am excited to present you with these easy, rewarding, and effective recipes. Power does live in your pantry.

DEBORAH BURNES
Sebastopol, California

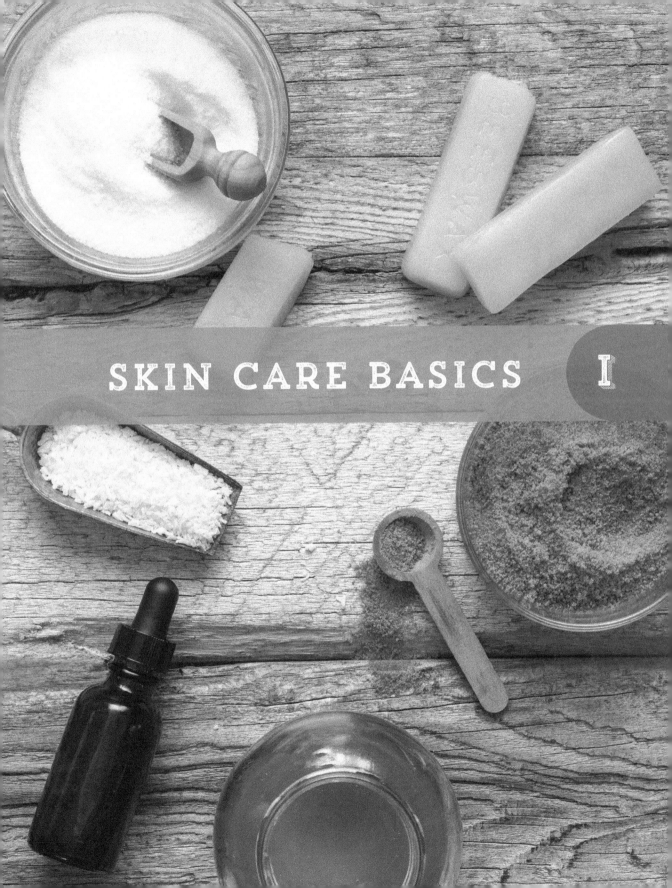

SKIN CARE BASICS   I

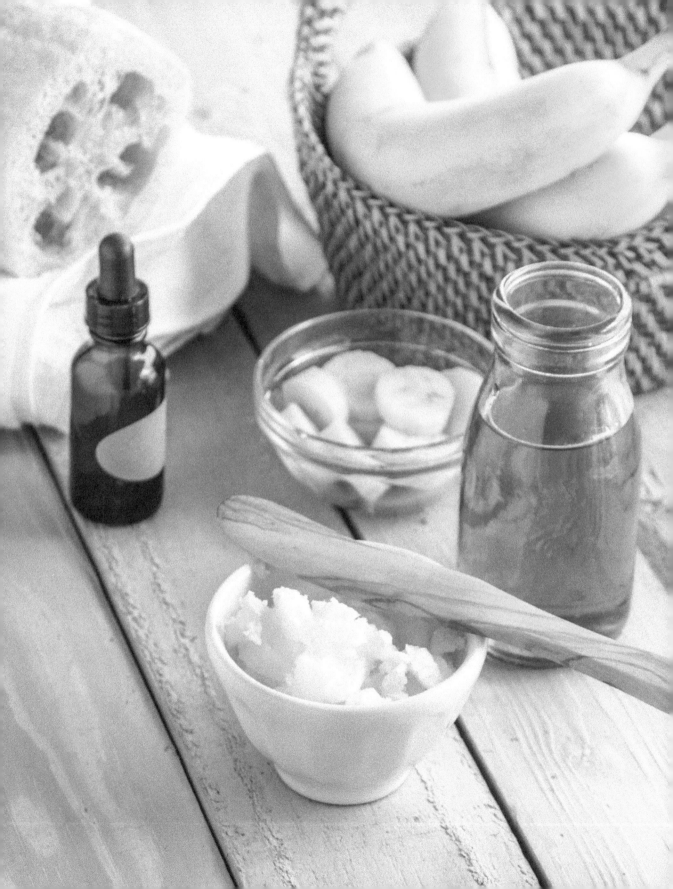

1

THE SKIN
YOU'RE IN

Skin is amazing. It is our largest organ, covering about 18–22 square feet of the average-size adult. Our skin literally holds us together and provides a barrier between our insides and the outside world. It's the first line of defense against pollutants, illness, and disease, making the health of your skin a priority for overall health. While it does protect us, skin also absorbs what it's exposed to into the bloodstream—like some of the toxic ingredients in skin-care products. That's why healthy skin is so essential for looking and feeling great.

The outer layer of skin, called the epidermis, is continually replacing itself with cells from the layer beneath it. This process is one of the key elements to keeping skin looking youthful. As we age, the renewal process slows, but it doesn't stop. We can help it along. For example, exfoliating daily with a good cleanser can enhance cell turnover and help maintain our skin's youthfulness. Unfortunately, in our sometimes crazy-busy lives, we often put daily skin matters at the bottom of our to-do lists. However, small steps each day can have a profound effect on keeping pores clear and restoring vitality to tired skin. Proper care can keep our skin healthier longer and slow the skin-damaging effects of the aging process.

When we scan the beauty aisle in search of products to help our skin, we may come across lots of lotions claiming to be the latest miracle in a jar. These products are often loaded with chemicals that may actually cause skin to age faster or exacerbate the problems they claim to fix. Magazine ads, featuring celebrities who never seem to age, urge us to run out and buy whatever cream promises to take 20 years off our skin—just like it did for the (photoshopped) spokesperson!

I've built my career on the fact that natural products can keep skin looking amazing, and even I occasionally get tempted to buy into the outlandish sales pitch. But I do know that these products and images aren't what they seem. This is just a reminder of how persistent and powerful these misleading messages can be.

I'm not claiming that a natural skin-care routine (or any skin-care routine, for that matter) can stop time—and nor would I want it to. Our laugh lines and wrinkles are signs of experience and part of the natural and inevitable process of aging. I love sharing what I know with my clients and helping them set realistic goals to find a routine that works for them. It's my hope that the advice and recipes in this book will empower you with the natural tips and tricks estheticians use, allowing you to create products and habits that garner the results you're seeking.

SKIN TYPES

Our skin can be a mirror for what's going on inside our bodies and can also reflect what it's exposed to in our environment. I've found that most of my clients have accurately assessed their skin type, and you likely have as well. While I find most self-assessments to be fairly accurate, I do have to remind people that skin type isn't a permanent marriage. It can change as we age or even over the course of a few months. Some women have dry skin for most of their lives, and then start to get a few oily patches here and there. Or some may relocate, and their new environments leave once-oily skin feeling parched. Being open to the fact that skin type can shift can help you adapt if changes occur. Sometimes skin can seem as unpredictable as life itself. Nevertheless, knowing your current skin type will help you create DIY products that will work best for you.

NORMAL

Normal skin is neither overly dry nor overly oily. Women with normal skin still deal with environmental concerns (like sun protection and air pollution), the occasional breakout, or normal aging. Even "normal" skin has issues that need attention. However, I often see people with normal skin reaching for products that are not appropriate for their needs. If you have a few blemishes, you don't need to switch to an entire acne-fighting regimen. You can simply spot treat the blemishes until they disappear.

I always encourage women to use products with active ingredients only if they need it; for example, when I see women in their twenties with beautiful, youthful skin applying a high-powered anti-wrinkle cream, I explain that they don't need these ingredients just yet. It's kind of like taking antibiotics when you're not sick. Not only won't the antibiotics work, but it's also possible to build a resistance to them. Skin can work the same way, so if we're using strong ingredients too soon, they may be less effective when we actually need them. With normal skin, the best strategy is to maintain healthy habits to preserve skin's youthfulness by protecting it from damage, spot treating problem areas, and restoring luster as needed.

DRY

Dry skin can exhibit slight scaliness, flakes, tightness, or be ashy, red, or rough. Dryness can result when the skin is lacking fluids (dehydration) or oils (moisture). You need a balance of both fluid and oil to have properly hydrated skin. There are many factors that contribute to dry skin—from constant exposure to low humidity, air conditioning, and heating in office buildings and homes to chemicals in skin-care products. Given that we're all exposed to some of these drying elements, there are steps everyone can take to help protect the skin from these agents, such as washing your face with lukewarm water (as opposed to hot), eating foods with omega-3 fatty acids (like flaxseed and nuts), and limiting dehydrating foods (like caffeine and alcohol).

Some skin-care products that aim to treat dry skin are filled with dehydrating chemicals or lack necessary ingredients for transdermal penetration (a substance's ability to get into your skin). This means that even though some women are regularly applying moisturizer in the morning and evening, they still experience dryness because the product they are using simply sits on top of the skin or is packed with moisture-robbing chemicals. If you battle with dry skin, switching to products with ingredients that will neither impart, nor rob, your skin of fluids and oils can provide you with relief from dry skin.

OILY

Oily skin is not necessarily oily all the time; it often makes its presence well known around midday with shiny patches on the nose, forehead, or chin. People with oily skin might experience frequent breakouts due to an excess of sebum (an oily secretion produced by the sebaceous glands) that mixes with dead skin cells and causes a plug in the pores. Bacteria that can live on your skin thrive in the excess oil in your pores. Keeping congested pores clean is a top priority to help the skin function properly and reduce oil production.

We've all heard cosmetic companies touting the importance of using oil-free products, but I'll let you in on a little secret: oil on oil actually stops the skin's overproduction of oil. However, when it comes to your skin, not all oils are created equal. You want to use oils that are non-comedogenic (meaning they don't clog pores) and will help your skin balance and maintain normal oil flow. Jojoba oil (which is actually a wax that closely resembles your skin's sebum) is a perfect example—it can be used to help rebalance the skin, assist with oil regulation, and keep the pores clear. I recommend steering clear of oil-free products, which seem like the perfect fix for an oily complexion, but they can instead dry out your skin and lead to increased oil production. This might sound a bit crazy, but putting the right oil on your oily skin will actually reduce the overall oil and balance out your skin, and oily skin still needs moisture. So instead, look for products that rebalance oil production and keep pores clean. Here's a bit of good news: oily skin tends to age more slowly than dry skin.

COMBINATION

Combination skin can be dry on the cheeks and oilier in the "T" zone (the forehead, nose, and chin), presenting challenges that are common in both skin types. Women with combination skin are often unsure how to care for their complexion, as it can be unclear which products will

best suit them. There are several approaches for combination skin. You can use a serum (a skin-care product targeted to a specific issue) only on the area where the skin is having an issue. You don't need to treat all your skin with the same active ingredients. Or you can work on cleaning and unclogging your pores. Oftentimes, women will develop combination skin with weather changes, or through hormonal changes. By deep cleaning your pores, balancing your pH, and proper oil and hydration balance, some women find this the effective solution to restoring a unified skin type. Other women will always have a bit of excessive dryness in one area or excessive oil in the T-zone; for them, the deep cleaning will help along with spot treating the problem area with different products.

A facial oil, such as jojoba oil, can moisturize dry areas while bringing balance to oily zones. This makes it the perfect choice for both oily and dry skin. Choose an oil that also has skin-loving ingredients, like carrot oil (which is high in vitamin A) and rose hip oil (which is high in vitamin C). Additionally, using a pH-balancing toner, like the Tea and Vinegar Detox Toner (page 69), can keep dead skin cells turning over and prevent clogged pores.

DAILY DAMAGE

From car exhaust fumes to cold viruses, our skin is constantly being challenged. Taking care of our skin and reducing the exposure burden is crucial if we want to stay as healthy as possible. Knowing the different sources of damage is an important first step in protecting our skin so that our skin, in turn, can protect us.

CHEMICALS IN SKIN-CARE PRODUCTS

The average American slathers on or lathers up with eight personal-care products every day. Just this seemingly harmless combination of deodorant, toothpaste, soap, shampoo, and lotions exposes us to about 138 chemicals daily. That is a huge burden for the skin and body to absorb. The thought of changing your entire routine and letting go of all your favorite products can leave a person paralyzed. Although it is a great idea to switch chemical-laden products with natural-ingredient counterparts, there is no need to feel that you have to switch everything. Start slowly and do what is easy and feels right for you. Even a small reduction will lessen the load.

Rather than aiming for perfection, and driving yourself crazy, it's fine to take steps to reduce some of the chemical exposure. I always discuss deal breakers with my clients. What products can't they live without? We make two piles of their everyday products. One pile is "can live without," and the other is the "have to have" pile. When we go through this process, it's surprising to my clients how many products they can actually live without! Then, I offer swaps for the "have to have" pile, like the ones you'll find in the DIY recipes in this book.

The pile of toxic "have to haves" shrinks quickly. This can happen for you, too, when you begin to make changes in the products you use daily. Start with the ones you have the most exposure to (for example, those you soak in or apply all over your body, as opposed to a product you'll wash off or one that covers little surface area). Then consider the alternatives and try them out.

POOR NUTRITION

What we put into our bodies can certainly affect our skin, so we want to take steps to avoid foods that are going to put a burden on our organs. Foods and beverages such as alcohol,

SMOOTHING OUT ROUGH PATCHES

If there's one part of the body that feels the impact of our busy lives, it's our feet—literally. They support us all day, every day, and often get jammed into tight boots in the winter and exposed to dirt and elements in summer. Giving your tootsies a little pampering can go a long way to relax your entire body and nourish those soles. At my spa we often begin treatments with a foot soak. It is amazing how you can see someone completely relax from head to toe by just soaking their feet. The shoulders and jaw drop and their eyes start to close. Remember everywhere you go, your feet get you there! On one of those days where you are over exhausted and overstressed, try relaxing feet first.

For the ultimate in quick relaxation, try the Tea Tree Foot Soak on page 164 and follow up with a rubdown of body butter or a spritz of neroli hydrosol (a sweet distillation of orange blossoms, which helps ease tension). It's incredible how much five minutes can pay off when it comes to resetting the entire body.

caffeine, sugar, and white flour can be dehydrating and have negative effects on skin, as well as highly processed foods, fast food, and not having enough variety in your diet to supply the needed nutrients for glowing healthy skin and hair. Try adding dark leafy greens, fruits, and vegetables as well as flaxseed, chia seeds, nuts, seeds, herbal teas, and whole grains to your diet. Eating as close to the source is one of the best healthy skin diets.

That said, life is just too short to skip what I call vitamin J (aka "vitamin junk"—those little items that bring us happiness, but aren't necessarily loaded with nutrients). When it comes to vitamin J, it's not just about the food; it's whatever we know isn't healthy for us but we choose to indulge in anyway. For me it is not the vitamin J that concerns me, it is making sure you are educated so you are consciously choosing your poisons, not letting them choose you. Having said that, I like to live by what I call the 85/15 percent rule. Eighty-five percent of the time, I try to do what is best for my body and health. Fifteen percent of the time, I indulge in my version of vitamin J. You might find a 90/10 or a 50/50 lifestyle works best for you.

HARSH EXFOLIANTS

Scrubbing our skin can feel so satisfying; it's like our minds know that our bodies are sloughing off dead cells and impurities to revel a fresh, new state. Some exfoliators, though, can cause microdermabrasions (little tears that damage and age the skin). Avoid ingredients like apricot kernels and walnut hulls. No mattered how powdered they seem, they'll still have jagged edges, which will scratch the skin. Unlike sugar or salt, which dissolve and get smaller, walnut shells and apricot kernels stay hard, as they do not dissolve in water. When I was a kid growing up in New York City, we used to scrape apricot pits on the sidewalk after we ate the fruit. (I don't remember why we did this, but the memory is vivid!) Those kernels were so hard that they never seemed to grind down. The same is true when they scrape against the skin.

When looking for exfoliators, choose those with ingredients that are round (have no jagged edges), are dissolvable in water, and/or absorb dead skin cells. Gentle exfoliators that absorb dead cells are a wonderful alternative to the tougher scrubs. Goat milk and apple cider vinegar are two ingredients that help skin cells turn over without causing damage. If you love the feeling of scrubbing, salt and sugar can be great for your body. On the face, I like to use mild exfoliators, such as almond meal, quinoa flour, and ground sunflower seeds. Try the Quinoa Cleanser (page 53) or Detox Cleanser (page 56), which leave behind essential fatty acids in addition to buffing.

SUN EXPOSURE

There's no shortage of scientific evidence about the role UV light plays in skin damage. Sunscreen seems like the obvious solution for protecting the skin from these damaging rays and preserving the youthfulness of your complexion. But sunscreen is one of the biggest toxic chemical culprits, which leaves very few options for proper sun protection. The good news is: there are more natural brands of sunscreen emerging. Beyond wearing sunscreen free of toxic chemicals, if I know I'm going to be out in the sun for an extended period of time, I practice what I call sun avoidance. I wear big sunglasses with UVA/UVB protection lenses along with a hat and long, thin layers to cover my arms and legs. Whenever possible, I seek out the shade. If I know that I have to be out for an extended period and I cannot avoid the sun, I will use whichever sunscreen I can find with the fewest toxic chemicals.

BACTERIA

Treating your skin gently (for example, not picking at your skin or using makeup brushes that haven't been cleaned in a while) is important for keeping bacteria off your face. Picking and self-extraction of blackheads can traumatize skin, causing capillaries to burst, or even cause scarring, in addition to allowing bacteria to enter or spread. Other ways we unknowingly expose our skin to bacteria and oils that can cause breakouts is through hair on our face (such as bangs) as well as our everyday items, like hats and cell phones, which get exposed to countless microorganisms, as well as skin oil. Making little changes, such as using headphones with your cell phone, regularly cleaning the surface of your phone, or seeing an esthetician instead of attempting self-extraction, can keep bacteria off your skin. If you're prone to breakouts or oily skin, it is a good idea to change your pillowcase often, keep your hair off your face, and avoid scarves, hats, and headbands if you are developing blemishes under and around the areas they cover. I have worked with

professional football players who had a terrible time with acne at the helmet line. If you cannot get rid of the culprit (football players need those helmets!), make sure you clean your skin and the surface that touches your skin before and after using. Proper daily skin care and working with an esthetician will help maintain your skin and keep it (mostly) bad bacteria free.

STRESS

The way our skin looks and feels is affected by everything from our sleep to our stress levels. While it can be impossible at times to walk away from stress and business (or our many commitments at work, home, and in the community), there are some simple techniques that can bring a sense of calm to the day. Breathe. It can help improve how we feel in stressful moments, which can have an impact on the entire day. I encourage my clients to start and finish their day with three deep breaths. I find this is something everyone can make time for, and the couple of minutes it takes will help start and end your day in a more balanced, refreshed, and regrouped way.

While lying in bed, place your hand on your belly. As you breathe in, feel your belly expand, and when you breathe out, contract; repeat. Some people like to think of a word or phrase while they breathe, like inhaling joy and exhaling happiness. Beyond morning and night, people often do these breathing exercises midday to feel centered during those crazy stressful moments. Try it.

Aromatherapy can also ease tension. Scents like neroli (which helps with anxiety), rose (for cranky moods), and lavender (for all-over stress reduction) can have a huge impact on your disposition. Some of the recipes include essential oils and hydrosols (flower water), providing aromatherapeutic benefits while you care for your skin. But aromatherapy can be as simple as dabbing a bit of an essential oil onto a hanky, stashing it your purse, and taking it out when you need to relax. When my girls were in school, I made them "study buddies." These were little kits containing various essential oil blends for them to open up when they needed to de-stress during an exam. These kits became so popular that everyone asked to use them— including the teachers. I have also used neroli and rose water spray on my children since they were little. Whenever one was in a cranky mood, I would spray a little rose hydrosol over her head; if one was feeling anxious, out came the neroli. Now even at 22 and 26, all I have to do is reach for the spray and their moods still shift.

YOUR IDEAL SKIN-CARE REGIMEN

Your healthiest skin is a marriage between you and your habits. While most of this book focuses on amazing recipes that address many of the skin concerns I hear about from women, I also wanted to share my daily recommendations with you. Consistency is key when it comes to skin health. It's kind of like flossing: at first, it seems impossible to fit into your oral hygiene routine, but once you do, it feels effortless and necessary. Good skin-care routines are the

NUTRITION FOR GREAT SKIN

Diet can affect our skin and energy levels. This is why I encourage people to drink more water, eat a "rainbow" of fruits and vegetables, and include foods with essential fatty acids in their diet. When I work with clients, I ask them to describe their daily diet. We then go over skin-loving foods (like leafy greens and foods rich in omega-3s fatty acids) and foods that are contraindicated for skin health. When we look over their usual choices, I'll ask what's on their not-so-good-for-the-skin list that they cannot live without (in other words, what are their deal breakers?). Some people might say, "I'm not going to give up my coffee, but I could carry a water bottle with me and sip water throughout the day." It is the small changes that add up to a big difference.

I also encourage people to make changes slowly. For example, consider having fewer cups of coffee and two more glasses of water each day. Eliminate two desserts per week and add one kale salad or a smoothie that includes flaxseeds or spinach. Change can be hard and there is no need to force yourself to do too much at once. Doing it slowly, over time is usually easier for everyone and feels more natural. I find the more you add healthy foods the more your body starts to crave them, making the process even smoother.

For skin health, start by looking at your usual diet and make some small changes to include more skin-loving foods and beverages and eliminate some of the less desirable ones.

same. You might not be used to all the pampering, but over time, it won't feel like an effort at all and will garner the results you are after. As with any marriage, it will take time to get into the groove. So when you first begin a new routine, be mindful that it may take an entire month for it to feel effortless and to see results.

CLEANSER

For the best results, cleanse your face morning and night. Smooth the product onto warm, damp skin with your middle and ring finger, working in circular motions. Pro tip: wash your face from the bottom up. This helps fight gravity and stimulates blood flow to skin cells. When caring for your face, always include your neck! Use warm water, never hot.

TONER

In the very beginning of my practice, I discovered that some of my clients were looking to save time and money by skipping the toner. "Toner is something you can skip," I'd tell them. I wish I could go back to each and every person I said that to and let them know how wrong I was. Toner might seem like an unnecessary step, but I assure you, this is far from the truth. It helps tighten pores and prep them for the day, rebalances your skin's pH level, and gets rid of any excess, oil, and dirt the cleanser may have left behind. Toner is so easy to make, and it's a great place to start when converting to a DIY routine. For the best results, use toner morning and night after cleansing.

SERUM

Think of serum as your problem solver. Serum is used to target skin concerns, like acne, wrinkles, or nutrient-depleted skin. If you are using serum, it should be applied twice a day, after cleansing and toning your skin and before your moisturizer. Let it settle in for a moment, and then apply the moisturizer over it. Since this a product that targets a specific skin condition, only add serum to your routine as needed. When you use a serum that's not called for, not only can it be a waste of money, but it can also be a waste of skin-healing actives (the active ingredients in the product). In other words, if you need the benefits of that active ingredient later, it might not be as effective if you used it all along.

MOISTURIZER

Hydration is critical to keeping skin youthful. To get the full effects of healthy, hydrated skin, you need to have a balance of oil and fluid. This balance will help restore cellular damage, allow for better transdermal penetration, and maintain vital nutrients. Regardless of skin type, everyone needs fluid and oil in their skin, which means women with oily skin can still be both dehydrated and lacking oil where your skin needs it. Without applying a moisturizer to oily skin, you can actually make matters worse. No matter the skin issues you face, oils can provide deep, penetrating hydration, so moisturizer is a must. For the best results, use moisturizers morning and night after toner (or serum, if you are using one).

MASKS

Masks are truly workhorses of a great skin-care system. Unfortunately, most of us are so busy that we just can't find the time to apply them—they seem like a once-a-year indulgence. However, I have a pro tip to make it easy to make masks part of your everyday routine. Not only that, the antiquated method of letting the mask dry on your skin isn't even good for your skin. The best place to apply a mask is while you are showering. It's like having your own personal esthetician in your home! By applying the mask in the shower, the warm steam helps draw the toxins and dirt out of your pores and pushes the active ingredients into your skin, right where you want them. It's that lovely push and pull of the warm, moist heat that makes your mask more powerful and effective.

STEAMS

A weekly facial steam prepared with skin-loving ingredients works double time, opening your pores to release trapped debris while allowing the beneficial properties in your steam mixture to penetrate deeply. The warm steam also increases the blood flow to your skin, which brings more oxygen to your skin's cells. It also stimulates perspiration, which further helps remove dead skin and other gunk. The ingredients you include in your steams can treat certain skin issues or just provide a wonderful general cleansing. The steams included in the recipe section make a great team; pick and choose among them as needed.

EVEN MORE ON MASKS

There are three key ways masks work: they can affect skin topically, mid-pore, or deep-pore. Topical masks can be used daily to treat fine lines or remove dead skin cells. Mid-pore masks prevent buildup in your pores and supply nutrients to your skin. These can be used three times a week and keep your pores in good shape. They can also keep your skin prepped for a deep-pore mask, which is where you really remove the buildup that comes from pollution, skin-care chemicals, smoke, makeup residue, rancid oils, and more. While deep-pore masks work wonders for clearing out your pores, you don't want to overuse them. I suggest everyone do a deep-pore mask once a week; however, depending on your lifestyle, you may need a deep-pore mask more or less often. Rotating between the three types of masks will make a world of difference for the health and radiance of your complexion.

FIVE REASONS TO DIY

It's hard to conceptualize all the toxic chemicals that are in our skin-care products. When a product comes in a beautiful tube and is labeled "organic oat honey and lavender body butter," it can be easy to think that it's good for us. The front of the label is often used to sell us what the brand thinks we want to hear, or what we're meant to believe, so we slather away unknowingly. When we look closer and read the actual ingredients, sadly we can see the all-natural and organic branding is not the real story. If we were given the same chemicals

TIPS FOR MAINTAINING HEALTHY HAIR

- Use a wide-tooth comb instead of a brush.
- Wait until your hair is dry before combing or brushing, except when applying conditioner.
- Reduce heat damage that comes from styling with irons, curlers, and blow dryers on high heat. Experiment with styles that don't require heat to find one you like.
- Comb or brush from the ends up.
- Use soft, loose ponytail holders for styles that need them. Never use rubber, which breaks hair and causes damage.
- Protect your hair from the elements by wearing a hat.
- Use silk or satin pillowcases.
- Trim your hair every six to eight weeks to keep ends healthy.
- Wash your hair less often and use warm, not hot, water.
- Don't towel dry your hair, because it's more fragile when wet. Instead, blot wet hair with a towel. There are towels on the market specifically made to dry hair quickly.
- Eat nutrient-rich foods that promote healthy skin and hair.
- Apply shampoo to scalp, and wash your scalp in small circular motions to increase blood flow.
- Gently squeeze out any excess water before applying conditioner.
- Apply conditioner and comb through with a wide-tooth comb.
- Clean your hairbrushes and combs regularly.

contained in that lotion in a shot glass, would we drink it? By taking control of what's in our products, we can swap out toxic chemicals in favor of ingredients that are beneficial to our skin and our overall health.

1. **You'll save money.** Walk into Sephora or Nordstrom, and you're bound to find "luxury" body scrubs selling for $30, $50, or even $70. A lot of those scrubs include a lengthy list of toxic chemicals on their label, which can cause skin damage. On the flipside, the scrub recipes in this book contain ingredients you might have at home or can easily buy in the grocery store and use for cooking, too. Pick up some avocado oil for the Basic Body Oil (page 104), and I bet you'll use it to dress salads as well. Mix a few of these oils to make a versatile body oil, stir in some used coffee grounds (they're more effective than unused ones), and add a little sea salt. You'll have a powerful cellulite-eliminating scrub that will save you a lot of money, and not take a lot of time.

2. **You control the quality.** Would you rather cook with a fresh, sweet, vine-ripened tomato or a canned one? How about indulging in store-bought cookies or warm chewy cookies from the oven? The same is true with skin-care products. A commercial product might tout certain ingredients on

its label, but it's hard to know if they used a high-end, organic, and fresh version of the ingredients, or an old or cheaper version. And without having access to their formula you can't know how much of this ingredient is actually contained within the product. When you're making your products at home, you're in charge of everything that goes into the jar and in what quantities.

3. **You'll know the products are at their peak.** The longer a product sits on the store shelf, the less effective it will be. When you're creating your own products, you'll know exactly when it was packaged and how long it should last. Ingredients have an expiration date, and if you use them when they're fresh, you can use less and get more out of them.

4. **You'll be helping the environment.** Mass-produced body products contribute to pollution with chemicals when they're being manufactured and are then packaged in plastic and, oftentimes, boxed up in cardboard. A large number of these products will go unused or wind up down the drain when you wash them off, further adding to their toxic effect on the environment. I call it the triple threat. First, during manufacturing, the chemicals pollute the environment, then they pollute our bodies when we use them, and finally, they pollute the environment again when they go down the drain.

5. **You can make DIY products into great gifts.** When my daughters were school-aged, we loved to make bath bombs and scrubs for their friends and teachers. It was amazing to me how in demand our home-made products became around holiday time. Everyone appreciates a gift made from the heart, and natural beauty products really show the love.

BATH BOMB MASTERY

To ensure you get the best outcome every time you make a bath bomb, follow these steps:

Combine baking soda and citric acid in a glass or metal bowl (do *not* use wood when making bath bombs) and mix well.

If you are using any additional powders or petals (milk, lavender), add to the bowl and mix again.

If butters are incorporated into your bath bomb, heat until just melted but not scorching hot. Be very careful, as heated butters can burn the skin and cause blisters. If the butter is too hot, let it cool down before using. When the butter is still melted and warm, mix it in with the dry ingredients with a spoon or your hands.

If you are not using butters in your bath bomb:

Add the essential oils, mix with your hands, and wet the mixture with one spray of vodka one at a time. The mixture should start to come together and feel slightly "sticky" in your hands. Continue spraying one quick squirt of vodka at a time into the mixture until it feels sticky and cold when it starts to form (fizzers that do incorporate butters will use less vodka to form).

When the batter is ready, press it firmly into the bottom of your molds (Teflon baking molds work great. They come in a muffin shape; when filled only three-quarters full, they make a nice shape. Any hard plastic mold will work as well). Let dry overnight; then turn the bath bomb out of the mold and use it in the tub.

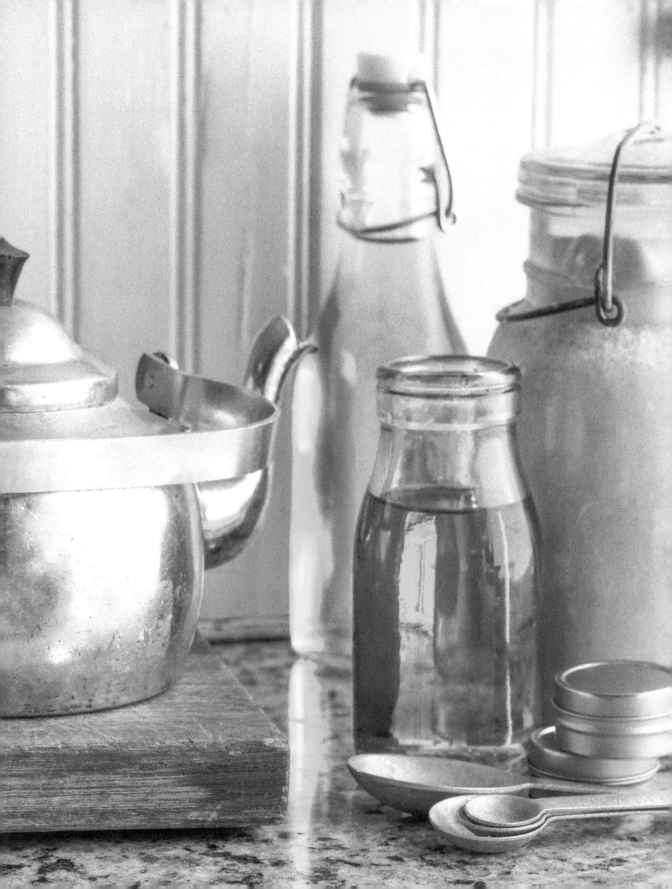

2

STOCKING UP & GETTING PREPARED

Some people think natural products aren't as effective as conventional ones. This couldn't be less true; when formulated correctly, natural products are incredibly effective. Nature's powerful bounty offers an array of skin-loving benefits. Oftentimes, we don't even think about how powerful the foods we eat can be when used for our skin and hair. For example, olive oil can be used right from the bottle as a skin-hydrating makeup remover, and strawberries and oatmeal make a gentle, vitamin-packed cleanser.

What I love most about creating homemade natural beauty products is how easy it is. You can whip up luxurious masks, foot soaks, and body butters using ingredients in your pantry and some basic tools from your kitchen. It's so simple that you can make natural beauty products virtually anywhere, including in a hotel room. If I'm traveling and I forget to bring a product with me or if I run out, a quick trip to the breakfast buffet has pretty much everything I need. For a DIY mask, for example, I gather some oatmeal, bananas, coffee, and a little yogurt and prepare the mask in my room. It's great for helping ease travel-related stress, dehydration, and puffy eyes.

I adore fresh ingredients, and simple straightforward skin-care products are easy and inexpensive to make—for yourself, to give as gifts, with your kids, or during a girls' night in. When my daughters were young, I was always looking for fun, creative birthday party ideas. Hosting DIY nights became the thing to do at our house. After a make-your-own pizza dinner activity, we'd craft our own personal skin-loving treatments with a bevy of odds and ends (avocado, buttermilk, clay, and so on). Then, we'd all do facial masks. The girls always had a blast.

This chapter offers a list of tools you'll need to succeed and some of my favorite natural ingredients that can transform and heal your skin in incredible ways. While many ingredients can be found in the grocery store, other products like certain clays or oils are most readily available from various online retailers and specialty stores. There is no need to run out and grab everything on the list; simple swaps of one ingredient for another can be made—such as soymilk in place of goat milk.

TOOLS OF THE TRADE

This section lists all the kitchen tools I find helpful for making products at home. While the list might look lengthy, most of the recipes I share in this book can be prepared using little more than cupboard staples, like bowls, spoons, and glass containers. In most cases, if you don't have an item, you can swap one tool for another. So don't feel as if you need a kitchen makeover before getting started.

PREPARATION EQUIPMENT

I'm an avid baker, and baking is known for being a precise art. As with baking, having better tools makes the process easier, but it isn't essential for a good product. Since the recipes I share in this book are meant to be made at home, wherever possible I've kept the equipment you'll need to prepare your DIY skin-care products to the basics. There are plenty recipes in the book though, so if something calls for a tool you don't have on hand, try a different recipe with similar benefits that includes tools you do have.

To make your DIY products, you can use your regular cooking tools and vessels—except when it comes to making products that contain beeswax. Though beeswax is a wonderful ingredient in body butters and lip balms, it can be impossible to completely remove it from your kitchen implements. So, if you're using beeswax in your recipes, set aside some kitchen tools just for your lovely beeswax beauty products.

- Bowls
- Cheesecloth, nut milk bag, or small strainer
- Grater
- Measuring cups
- Pots
- Spatulas
- Spoons

When making your own products, be sure to use nonporous utensils, preferably stainless steel. Because wooden utensils are porous, they can "hold" contaminants such as mold, bacteria, and fungus, which can then contaminate your products. I also prefer glass, enamel, or stainless steel bowls to their plastic counterparts when making products, but especially for storage. Some recipes call for a hot infusion, which involves steeping herbs or tea; a cheesecloth, nut bag, or small strainer will allow you to easily strain those infusions and add nutrient-packed waters to your skin-care products. Some ingredients need to be grated, so that's where your grater will come in handy. Measuring cups allow you to carefully measure out your ingredients so that nothing goes to waste.

USED FREQUENTLY

- Funnels
- Hand mixer or stand mixer
- Ice trays
- Mini food processor or coffee grinder
- Nonlatex surgical gloves
- Whisk

A mini food processor or coffee grinder helps pulverize ingredients, such as strawberries and avocados that tend to stay chunky when chopped by hand and stirred with a spoon.

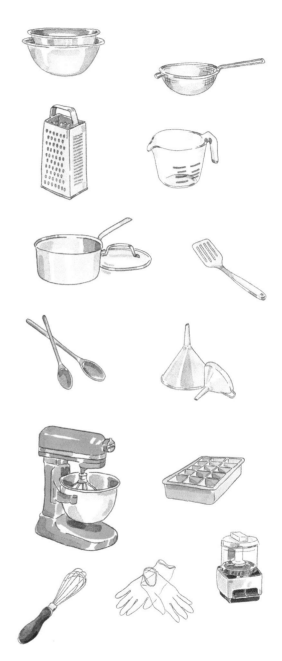

Clockwise from top: bowls, small strainer, measuring cup, spatula, funnels, ice tray, mini food processor, nonlatex gloves, whisk, stand mixer, spoons, pot, grater

Because of the small quantities often used in this book, a full-size food processor would be too big for your purposes. A whisk is perfect for beating a single egg white when called for in a recipe, but a hand mixer can be used as well. A funnel is sometimes necessary for pouring your product into a container with a small opening, ice trays are perfect for freezing small amounts of a product for later use, and surgical gloves will keep your hands clean, if you prefer, while you are having fun!

USED OCCASIONALLY

- Mini slow cooker (1½ quarts or 20 ounces), or a double boiler
- Silicone or Teflon molds

Some of the recipes call for a mini slow cooker (or, as an alternative, a double boiler). This item will help make your DIY life easier, especially if you love working with beeswax. (Remember, though, you'll need a mini slow cooker just for your beeswax products.) Meanwhile, silicone or Teflon molds will shape your bath bombs. This is a little ironic because one of my rants is against silicone—it can clog your pores when included in skin-care products—but we are not applying it to our skin here, just using it as a tool, and we won't be storing any products in it, either.

STORAGE EQUIPMENT

I love to make the whole DIY process clean and green, so I reuse old jars to store my homemade products. You can save money and help the environment by doing the same. Instead of throwing used glass jars into the recycle bin—peel off labels, clean them well, and store them for later use. Other storage items include the following:

- Adhesive labels
- Decorative bottles and jars
- Mason jars
- Perfume rollers and/or atomizers
- Spray bottles
- Toner bottles

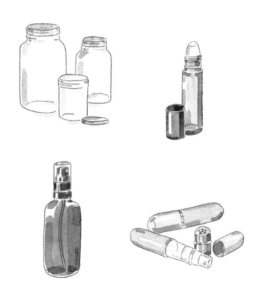

Left: double boiler, silicone molds; Above (clockwise): mason jars, perfume roller, atomizers, spray bottle

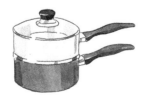

Atomizers and spray bottles are especially handy if you're planning to make perfumes, toners, and hairsprays. Shower-safe pump or squeeze bottles are perfect for shampoos and conditioners. For body butters, low-profile jars are best for ease of use. Using decorative bottles or jars for your DIY products can make your handiwork into wonderful gifts. Craft stores are great for finding beautiful glass jars to hold bath salts. For gift giving and even your own purposes, you can label the bottles with adhesive stickers. Creating and printing your own unique labels for your DIY products are a sweet touch for wedding and shower favors, or whenever gifting your DIY products.

APPLICATION TOOLS

I'm a tactile person and love applying products with my hands. DIY facial massages are a phenomenal way to get blood flowing. Even just applying a product to your face with your fingertips stimulates circulation. Nevertheless, your hands aren't your only choice. You can use:

- Cotton or silk washcloths
- Natural bristle fan brush

Soft all-cotton or silk washcloths are gentle enough to use on your skin and can make it easier to apply a full-body scrub. If you don't want to apply a face mask with your hands, a

SLOW COOKER OR CROCK-POT®—WHAT'S THE DIFFERENCE?

Many people use "Crock-Pot" instead of "slow cooker," and the two terms have come to have the same meaning. But there is a difference. Crock-Pot is the registered trademark of the Rival Company, which released the slow cooker in 1970. So while every Crock-Pot is a slow cooker, not every slow cooker is a Crock-Pot. Crock-Pots have heating elements on the bottom and sides, but other slow cookers usually have them only on the bottom. This book sticks to the term "slow cooker," but the recipes will work using any slow cooker or Crock-Pot.

A QUICK ALTERNATIVE TO THE STOVETOP

Butter, beeswax, and some oils require melting to properly incorporate them into your products. Beeswax is generally heated in a slow cooker or double boiler, while butters and oils are melted on the stovetop over low heat. However, if you're in a hurry, the microwave will do in a pinch. Always use appropriately sized, microwave-safe glass containers. When melting your beeswax in the microwave, be sure to use a container that you've dedicated to your beeswax products. It is best to microwave in 10-second intervals so that the wax, butter, or oil does not get hot enough to cause burns, or overheat. Overheating can cause discoloration and affect the efficacy of the ingredients. If you accidentally overheat your wax, butter, or oil, let it cool down a bit in the microwave before removing.

clean fan brush can be used instead. After you're done with your treatment, thoroughly cleanse the brush with a natural soap, rinse it completely, and then dry it with a blow dryer on a low setting. Rubbing alcohol can also be applied. This important process will extend the life of your brush and ensure that you're not sweeping any bacteria or built-up product onto your skin during the next application. Make sure to wash your washcloth after every use as well.

DIY RESPONSIBLY

When considering if a certain recipe is right for you, always consult with your doctor. If you have questions about any of the ingredients used in that product, if you are pregnant, or if you have a serious skin condition, getting your doctor's advice is essential. Also, always clean and sterilize your tools and test for any allergens to ensure you're making and using your products in the safest way possible.

CLEANSING TOOLS

Clean tools make effective, germ-free products. Use natural soap and clean dishrags to wash your kitchen tools and appliances, including new ones. Rinse them with water, making sure all the soap is washed away, and allow them to dry completely before using them in your DIY recipes or storing them away. For an extra but important measure, follow up by spraying a light mist of rubbing alcohol and letting it dry.

STERILIZING TOOLS

To sterilize my tools prior to use (following a thorough cleansing), I lay out plastic wrap so they do not get contaminated again and use rubbing alcohol in a spray bottle to spray down anything I'm going to use. Then, I allow the sterilized tools to dry on the plastic wrap (it happens pretty quickly and if there is a little dampness from alcohol, it won't contaminate your product the way water would). New jars and bowls may seem like they're ready to use right out of the package, but they may be treated with a chemical finish, so it's important to clean and sterilize those as well. If you have a dishwasher with a sanitary cycle, you can prep them in there.

During the process of making the products, it's important to keep all implements clean and dry. I lay spoons and utensils on a fresh piece plastic wrap or wax paper so I know they'll be resting on a clean surface until I need them again. It is extremely important to make sure there is no water (not even a droplet) on any utensils, bowls, or even your hands. Water can contaminate your entire batch and cause it to mold. When it's time to use your products, do not use damp or wet hands, use a sanitized utensil.

PATCH TESTING & ALLERGIES

Foods applied topically to skin may react differently than when they are ingested. For example, I love eating strawberries and do so regularly, but if I put pure strawberry jam on my face, my skin turns red and burns. So, with any new recipe, I recommend applying a dime-size amount of the product on your inner wrist before applying it to your face or body. Leave it on for 15 minutes, and then rinse it off. If your skin turns red or reacts in any way, you know there is something in that product that doesn't agree with your skin. To isolate and eliminate the disagreeable ingredient, try this same patch test with each of the ingredients used in the product you tested. You can do this for each ingredient *before* preparing the recipe, as well. If you know you have a skin allergy to a specific ingredient, you can swap out that ingredient for one that has similar benefits. Just because something is natural does not always mean it is right for you.

YOUR BEAUTIFUL PANTRY

The natural ingredients you'll read about here contain an array of skin-loving vitamins, minerals, acids, and more. Some are foods we commonly eat, while others are oils that have been pressed from various parts of plants. As with the tools of the trade, many of these ingredients can be found at your local grocery, in a health food store, or online. Before going out and buying everything listed in this chapter, peruse the recipes and choose a couple you'd like to begin with, then gather the ingredients you'll need.

PLANT-BASED PRODUCTS

Nature has been growing an abundant pharmacy for millennia, and the plant products called for in these recipes certainly prove this to be true. In general, I use organic flowers, teas, nuts, and herbs whenever possible. I feel organic is the best, but I'd rather you make a product with conventional ingredients than skip the recipe just because you don't have the organic variety.

ALFALFA. This nutrient-rich plant is beneficial for all parts of the body, including the skin. The chlorophyll it contains helps rid the body of impurities. It's also rich in vitamin A and enzymes (molecules that enhance biological processes).

ALMONDS. Almonds are loaded with antioxidants, which help slow the skin's natural aging process. They also contain omega-3 fatty acids, which are believed to reduce inflammation. Ground-up almonds (aka almond meal) are gentle exfoliators that won't cause microdermabrasions (little tears that damage and age the skin). I also make homemade almond milk, which is high in vitamins and protein, and use it in masks and facial cleansers. Store-bought almond milk can contain other ingredients that aren't necessary to the recipe you are making. If you can find pure almond milk without additives, feel free to use it.

ALOE VERA. The aloe vera plant contains more than 75 different nutrients, including beta-carotene, which can help with skin renewal. Called the "plant of immortality" by the ancient Egyptians, it stimulates the regeneration of skin cells. It contains lots of skin-loving amino acids (the building blocks of protein), which can help smooth fine lines and improve elasticity. I use gel, juice, or jelly depending on the recipe and desired consistency.

APPLE CIDER VINEGAR. Apple cider vinegar packs a powerful amount of alpha hydroxy acids—even more than most products that tout this ingredient on their labels. Alpha hydroxy acids are a group of compounds that are often added to skin-care products to help remove dead skin cells. But with apple cider vinegar, those acids are delivered to your skin from a natural source, making them alive, active, and more powerful. Apple cider vinegar also has antifungal properties, which is great for acne-prone skin and aids in reducing pore congestion. Apple cider vinegar also helps balance the pH level of skin, helping the skin to be neither too dry nor too oily.

APPLE JUICE. Apples are full of beneficial vitamins and compounds, and apple juice contains antioxidants derived from the skin and flesh of the fruit. The juice promotes circulation, which helps replenish old and damaged skin cells. The most important aspect to apple juice is malic acid, a natural form of alpha hydroxy acid.

APRICOT. This antioxidant-packed little fruit is a skin-care powerhouse. The vitamin A found in apricots helps repair skin damage. It also has anti-inflammatory properties.

ARROWROOT. A starch derived from the roots of various plants, arrowroot is a natural thickening agent. Aside from its ability to thicken your products, it can also help with transdermal penetration, which means that it helps active ingredients sink deeper into the skin.

AVOCADO. Avocado contains antioxidants, which protect the skin from environmental damage. It's packed with vitamin C, which is essential for the creation of collagen and elastin, and vitamin E, which fights oxidative damage and can help protect the skin from ultraviolet rays. The essential fatty acids in avocado hydrates the skin—including the scalp—and can help repair damaged skin and fight signs of aging.

BAKING SODA. This powder, which is technically known as sodium bicarbonate, deep cleans nails and hair. It's also a popular ingredient in oral health care products, though there's debate whether or not it's good for everyday brushing.

BANANA. Bananas contain amino acids, potassium, lectin (a protein), zinc, and vitamins A, B, C, and E, all of which are beneficial for the skin. This popular fruit can be used for everything from moisturizing to anti-aging treatments. Its benefits aren't limited to placing mashed banana on the skin, of course; eating bananas can promote skin health from the inside out.

BANANA FLOUR. Just the like fruit from which it's derived, banana flour is loaded with potassium, an important electrolyte that helps maintain fluid balance in the skin. It's also a great gluten-free flour for baking.

BAY LEAF. Even the most casual chefs keep bay leaf around for seasoning soups and stews, but this antioxidant-packed herb can also help rejuvenate skin and prolong its youthfulness. Bay leaf has antiseptic properties that fight acne and encourage blood flow to the skin.

BILBERRY TEA. Bilberry fruit is commonly dried and made into a tea. Full of flavonoids and tannins, bilberry tea is known to increase circulation and reduce swelling.

BIRCH. Birch bark contains anti-inflammatory and antibacterial properties that can help relieve eczema and similar skin problems. Birch leaves have a history of use in treating rashes.

BLACK TEA. Chock-full of vitamins that are naturally beneficial to the body, black tea is anti-inflammatory, which can help reduce swelling in the skin. The tannins found in black tea serve to protect the skin from environmental damage, as well as fight bacteria that can cause skin problems. The tannins also increase circulation, which promotes skin regeneration. As with many teas, black tea is also full of antioxidants that fight oxidative damage.

BURDOCK ROOT. In Chinese medicine, burdock root is used to reduce internal heat (which is perceived as a toxic element in this ancient health-care approach) and for blood cleansing

and skin healing. It's also known for its skin and hair benefits due to its antioxidant properties.

CALENDULA. A member of the daisy family, calendula flowers have been used medicinally since ancient times. This plant contains anti-inflammatory properties, which makes it an excellent skin-soothing ingredient.

CHAMOMILE TEA. Chamomile is an anti-inflammatory. It is a wonderful ingredient for those dealing with eczema and rosacea. It's also full of flavonoids, which have been shown to reduce skin damage resulting from oxidation.

CHIA SEEDS. These small seeds are super high in omega-3 fatty acids, which nourish the skin and help improve its functions as a barrier to the outside world. They expand and soften in water, which creates a little pouch of hydration, making the seeds a soft exfoliant for the skin. (They're much better for you than those plastic beads that come in some body washes!) The oils in chia seeds improve the skin's natural barrier by keeping it hydrated, so it's also great for dry skin.

CINNAMON. This popular autumn spice brings blood to the surface of the skin. It has antioxidant properties that aid in skin softening and also help remove dead skin cells. Due to its antibacterial and antifungal properties, cinnamon can also help with skin infections. An important note: cinnamon can make you sun sensitive and cause redness and irritation if used in too high a concentration.

CITRIC ACID. Naturally found in citrus fruits, this acid is often used as a preservative. When used in skin-care recipes, it works to remove old layers of skin and clears the pores, so that dirt and oil can escape. Citric acid is available in powdered form, but it is also abundant in citrus peels, which is one of the reasons why some DIY products suggest using the rind.

COCOA POWDER. Caffeine and theobromine are naturally found in cocoa powder; these two plant chemicals can help break down fats and are believed to have draining properties, which helps reduce swelling and cellulite. Cocoa powder is also rich in anti-aging antioxidants.

COCONUT. From coconut milk to coconut butter, I use this healthy, tropical nut in various forms in the recipes in this book. Whenever a recipe calls for the meat of the coconut, I use shredded, unsweetened coconut. Shredded coconut is an excellent mild exfoliant. Coconut in general has antibacterial properties and includes essential fatty acids, which hydrate the skin.

COFFEE. The caffeine in coffee helps with firming, toning, and tightening the skin. Because it's what's called a "restrictor" (it reduces inflammation and swelling), it can be beneficial for relieving puffy eyes. When I'm staying in a hotel, I sometimes dab some coffee on a tissue and apply it on the delicate under-eye tissue to reduce sleep- and travel-related puffiness. When a recipe calls for coffee grounds in a scrub or cleanser, used grounds are best, since the hot water has already activated the most powerful ingredients in the beans. This makes them better for the skin than grounds straight from the bag and eliminates waste.

CRANBERRY. Acidic and antiseptic, cranberry is a good addition to treatments for oily skin. Rich in antioxidants, it helps fight the signs of aging.

These bitter berries are also loaded with vitamin C, which helps the body produce collagen to keep your skin healthy.

CUCUMBER. Cucumber flesh is mostly water, but it also contains ascorbic acid (vitamin C) and caffeic acid, both of which soothe skin irritations, reduce swelling, and prevent water retention, making them helpful in treating swollen eyes, dermatitis, and burns. Cucumber has the same pH level as the skin; using it helps restore the protective acid mantle (a slightly acidic film on the surface of this skin), which is imperative for keeping bacteria and other contaminants from being absorbed. Cucumbers also have hydrating, nourishing, and astringent properties.

DANDELION ROOT. A somewhat bitter-tasting herb, dandelion root is high in skin-loving vitamins A and C.

ELDERBERRIES. Not only are elderberries delicious, but they are also rich in flavonoids (a powerful antioxidant) and full of nutrients that fight aging and acne, and aid in detoxifying the skin.

ELDERFLOWER. The plant from which the elderberry grows is an equally effective skin-care ingredient. Elderflower water is most commonly used in skin-care products and contains a host of good-for-you vitamins, like vitamins A, B_1, and B_2, as well as the always necessary vitamin C. Elderflower fights oxidative damage and can even fade scars and blemishes.

FENUGREEK. This spice has a host of skin-healing properties. Filled with skin-loving essentials such as vitamin A, B_1, and K, plus calcium, zinc, and selenium; it is a spice not only good for cooking, but great for shoring up skin to battle acne, reduce inflammation, and work as an exfoliator. It even helps prevent sun damage.

GINGER. Ginger is antiseptic, which means it's good for healing skin issues like acne. Its antioxidant content helps rid the body of toxins that can cause premature aging. Ginger also helps tone the skin, boosts blood flow, is anti-inflammatory, and calms puffiness.

GINSENG. Ginseng is known for its ability to soften and moisturize skin. It is also rich in vitamins, minerals, and antioxidants.

GREEN TEA. Scientists have said the anti-oxidants in green tea are some of the most powerful in the world. These antioxidant compounds—specifically the polyphenols and flavonoids—help prevent damage to the skin such as formation of wrinkles and inflammation.

HEMP FLOUR. Hemp flour is made from ground hempseed, which is rich in essential fatty acids, amino acids, vitamins, and minerals, all of which are beneficial for skin health.

HORSETAIL EXTRACT. The extract from the horsetail plant has anti-inflammatory and antiseptic properties; it works to help the body repair and regenerate damaged skin cells. It also contains silica, which helps form collagen. It is beneficial for hair health, and can reduce split ends and help with growth and loss.

IRISH MOSS. This seaweed is high in vitamins A, C, E, and K, as well as amino acids, calcium, and zinc. It also produces mucilage, which gives a "slip" to skin-care products and is useful as a detangler.

JUNIPER BERRIES. Juniper berries are believed to have antibacterial and antiseptic properties; they are wonderful for acne-prone skin. Juniper berries also help balance and regulate skin and can be used for detoxing and deep cleaning.

LAVENDER. The scent of lavender induces relaxation. The buds of the plant have an astringent quality, making them useful for both cleansing and healing the skin.

LEMON. Lemon contains phytonutrients, which are skin-healthy chemicals derived from plants. Specifically, citrus fruit contains bioflavonoids that help the skin absorb vitamin C, which is a powerful antioxidant. The scent of lemon is also known to be uplifting.

LICORICE ROOT TEA. Applied to the skin, licorice tea is anti-inflammatory, soothing and moisturizing. It is effective for treating rosacea and psoriasis, and is used as a skin lightning agent.

LUCUMA POWDER. Made from the Peruvian fruit, lucuma, this powder is filled with skin-loving iron, niacin, calcium, and beta-carotene, making it a wonderful skin-care ingredient. Coconut sugar is an easy and effective replacement if lucuma powder isn't on hand.

MANGO. This tasty fruit is packed with vitamins A and C. It is also a good source of beta-carotene, which can help with acne. Its antioxidants protect the skin from oxidative damage and can help maintain the skin's youthful appearance.

MILK THISTLE. The active ingredient in this plant is silymarin, which is a natural antioxidant with detoxifying benefits. Some people find it helpful for psoriasis and eczema.

MINT. This herb contains vitamins A, B, and C, which keep the skin healthy and protected. It's also a source of salicylic acid, a key ingredient in OTC acne-fighting products. Its astringent qualities help cleanse the skin and also stimulate blood flow. However, if you have a tendency toward redness, avoid mint facial products, soaps, and lotions.

NEROLI. Derived from the blossom of the bitter orange tree, the scent of neroli is calming. When used in skin-care products, it can help reduce redness.

NETTLE OR STINGING NETTLE. When used in skin-care products, nettles are astringent and anti-inflammatory. They also are known to help with scalp problems, both oiliness and dandruff.

OATS/OAT FLOUR. Both whole oats and oat flour are anti-inflammatory and soothing. They are excellent for relieving skin injuries like poison ivy and insect bites and are full of proteins that fortify the skin. The polysaccharides in oats can help prevent dryness, while their fat content moisturizes the skin. The saponins in oats (or the soap-like foaming substance in many plants) are natural cleansers that gently purify the pores.

OAT STRAW. Oat straw can help relieve dry, itchy, and irritated skin due to its high gluten and mucilage content. It is also a concentrated source of skin-, nail-, and hair-loving silica.

OLIVE LEAF EXTRACT. While we know much about olive oil and its benefits on the skin and for the body, olive leaf extract is just as potent as its seedy counterpart. Containing antioxidants and the bioflavonoid luteolin, this extract fights free radicals (oxidative damage) and combats the aging process.

OREGANO. This fragrant herb has numerous skin benefits. It fights oxidative damage; kills bacteria, fungi, and viruses; and reduces inflammation.

ORRIS ROOT. Derived from the root of the iris flower, orris root is used to as a fixative (holds the scent) in scented products, as a gentle exfoliation, breath freshener, and for tooth whitening.

PAPAYA. Papaya is rich in antioxidants, papain, vitamin A, and carotene, all of which can boost skin health. It helps hydrate the skin while removing dead skin cells. The antioxidants found in the fruit help repair environmental damage.

PAPRIKA. This popular spice is both antibacterial and anti-inflammatory. It contains several vitamins, including A and E, which are essential for skin health.

PERSIMMON. Long recognized for its skin-improving benefits in traditional Chinese medicine, persimmons are rich in anti-aging antioxidants and other beneficial compounds. Persimmon can help control the overproduction of sebum, which leads to oily skin.

PINEAPPLE. This fruit contains vitamin C, and bromelian, a skin-softening enzyme that removes dead skin cells. Bromelian also stimulates the production of a collagen, helping the skin look and feel younger.

POLENTA. Polenta is an excellent addition to foot or body-care recipes for its exfoliating properties and vitamin-packed content.

PUMPKIN. Pumpkin is packed with fruit enzymes, alpha hydroxy acids, antioxidants, and zinc. This allows pumpkin to increase cell turnover, eliminate dead cells, brighten and smooth skin, combat acne, and prevent aging. Pumpkin also has the ability to penetrate the deeper layers of your skin and help other ingredients do the same.

PUMPKIN SEEDS. Pumpkin seeds are a powerhouse for the skin. They're full of lipids—fats that can keep the skin moisturized and protect it from particulates in the air. The oil from the seeds helps regulate sebum and is wonderful for oily skin as well as is high in vitamin E. When ground, pumpkin seeds make a gentle exfoliator.

QUINOA FLOUR. Quinoa flour is made from ground quinoa seeds, which are a rich source of amino acids, niacin, potassium, manganese, and vitamin E, to help promote skin and hair health. Notably, it promotes the production of collagen.

REISHI MUSHROOM. These mushrooms contain high levels of polysaccharides, which are responsible for the skin's natural ability to hydrate and retain water. Polysaccharides are also imperative for both skin repair and renewal.

RICE WINE VINEGAR. Rice wine vinegar is sometimes used interchangeably with apple cider vinegar, but it has a different amino acid profile and boosts the absorbent properties of other ingredients. It is also extremely softening and smoothing.

ROOIBOS TEA. This tea is rich in skin-healthy compounds like flavonoids, superoxide dismutase enzymes (necessary for the production of healthy skin cells); it is antibacterial and hypoallergenic. Additionally, rooibos has a wonderful soothing effect on acne-prone skin.

ROSE JELLY. A jelly made from the petals of roses, it is used for its high content of vitamin C, to control excess oil and unclog pores, and its astringent and antibacterial properties.

ROSEMARY. Rosemary is full of phytonutrients and antioxidants that defend against oxidative damage. It's also antiseptic, antibacterial, and anti-inflammatory, which makes it an excellent ingredient for combating various skin issues and for deep-pore cleaning and detoxing.

SLIPPERY ELM BARK. Best known for its healing properties, the inner bark of the slippery elm tree can be used to treat skin conditions from psoriasis to cold sores. Dried, powdered, and mixed with water, the inner bark promotes smooth, glowing skin.

ST. JOHN'S WORT TEA. Known for its wound-healing and skin-soothing abilities, St. John's wort is antibacterial and anti-inflammatory. Great for sensitive skin.

STRAWBERRIES. Strawberries are packed with vitamin C, antioxidants, salicylic acid, alpha hydroxy acids, and natural exfoliating ingredients, so they make for a powerful acne-fighting cleanser and anti-aging treatment.

SUNFLOWER SEEDS. Along with their anti-inflammatory and antibacterial properties, sunflower seeds are full of skin-loving vitamin E. When ground, they make a gentle exfoliator that moisturizes at the same time.

TURMERIC. Turmeric is a powerful antioxidant, is anti-inflammatory, and helps expel toxins.

It is also antiseptic and antibacterial, both of which are good for dealing with skin issues. It also helps reduce the appearance of wrinkles and balance oil production, making it an effective addition to skin-care products.

VANILLA BEAN. Vanilla beans, which smell simply delicious, contain anti-inflammatory and antioxidant compounds. They're also a great source of B vitamins and even have antibacterial properties.

WALNUTS. These tasty nuts are rich in essential fatty acids, and like other nuts and seeds, they can serve as a gentle, moisturizing exfoliator when ground and added to a cleanser.

WHITE TEA. White tea is the least processed among black, white, and green teas. Its high level of antioxidants combats oxidative damage, making it a powerful player in any anti-aging routine.

WHITE WILLOW BARK. This anti-inflammatory is known for its ability to help reduce pain. It also contains salicylic acid, which helps control acne and breakouts and removes debris from congested pores.

WHITE WINE VINEGAR. Made from grapes, wine vinegars contain antioxidants such as resveratrol. Use white wine vinegar as opposed to red wine vinegar to avoid color stains.

WITCH HAZEL. Witch hazel reduces redness, itching, and swelling and can also ease the sting of bug bites. Because it is both an astringent and antioxidant, it is wonderful on young skin that is dealing with acne as well as on mature skin to preserve youthfulness and eliminate fine lines. The type of witch hazel found in pharmacies often contains alcohol. The recipes in this book call for pure witch hazel hydrosol.

WOLFBERRIES. Also known as goji berries, wolfberries are loaded with antioxidants and beta-carotene as well as skin-loving vitamin C.

OILS & MILKS

The hydrators of your pantry, oils and milks can be mixed together to make luxurious moisturizers and cleansers and are an essential component to your beauty pantry.

APRICOT OIL. High in essential fatty acids, apricot oil is a gentle oil that is great for both aging and sensitive skin.

ARGAN OIL. Rich in vitamins A and E, essential fatty acids, antioxidants, and squalane, which fights the degeneration of skin.

AVOCADO OIL. Due to its high levels of antioxidants and vitamins, avocado oil is wonderful for people with sun-damaged or dehydrated skin. It's easily absorbed deep into the skin and contains essential fatty acids, which can help nourish the skin.

BLACK CUMIN OIL. Black cumin oil is pressed from the seeds of a flowering plant native to Asia called *Nigella sativa*. Rich in various vitamins, minerals, essential fatty acids, and bioflavonoids, this oil is great for relieving redness, rejuvenating the skin, and fighting infection.

BUTTERMILK. The high lactic acid content in buttermilk, which is in its powdered form too, makes it an excellent exfoliator and skin softener.

The added bonus of the exfoliating properties of lactic acid is that it also helps brighten the skin.

CAMELLIA OIL. Derived from the seeds of the tea plant, camellia oil is high in vitamins and fatty acids. It's hydrating and rich in antioxidants, which help keep the skin looking youthful.

CARRIER OIL. This is the base oil to which an essential oil is added. Just a few drops of certain oils, such as rose hip and carrot oil, can be quite powerful, as well as expensive. Therefore, when formulating products, essential oils are often diluted in a carrier oil , like jojoba, sesame, or sunflower, both to extend the amount of the oil and avoid overpowering the product.

CARROT OIL. Carrot oil is rich in beta-carotene, which can help reduce sun damage. The vitamin A it contains can be used to maintain elasticity and clear up mild to moderate acne. Because the oil has emollient properties, it can help soften skin as well.

CASTOR OIL. Castor oil is both anti-inflammatory and antibacterial. Because of its ability to deeply penetrate into the skin, it makes a wonderful moisturizer and skin conditioner.

COCONUT MILK. Coconut milk is an intense hydrator for skin. It is also filled with essential fatty acids, including lauric acid, which is a known cleansing agent. Its vitamin C and copper content can help with fine lines and improve skin elasticity. There are a few different varieties of coconut milk in the grocery store, but the type I prefer for skin and hair treatments comes in a cardboard container and is found in the refrigerated section of the store.

COCONUT OIL. Coconut oil is antimicrobial, antifungal, antiseptic, and antibacterial properties. Just like all the other coconut-derived ingredients listed here, its benefits to the skin are numerous.

COMFREY LEAF OIL. The oil derived from the comfrey leaf is high in allantoin, which encourages the growth of new cells and reduces inflammation.

ESSENTIAL OILS. Derived from various parts of plants, pure essential oils add natural fragrance to your products, and can be used as an active ingredient in a product. Remember, although essential oils are natural, they can be caustic if overused, so use them sparingly and only the amounts called for in the recipes. Some common essential oils you'll encounter in the DIY products include bergamot, cardamom, cedar, cinnamon, cinnamon bark, clove, grapefruit, lavender, lemon, marjoram, myrrh, orange, patchouli, peppermint, rosemary, sage, sweet orange, tangerine, and tea tree.

GOAT MILK. Goat milk contains alpha hydroxy acids, which absorb dead skin cells and can help prevent fine lines. Because the fat molecules in goat milk are so small, it penetrates the skin and hydrates deeply. Goat milk has a pH level that's similar to our skin's pH level, making it gentle enough for almost everyone.

HEMPSEED OIL. Hemp is rich in omega 6 and omega 3 fatty acids, as well as linolenic acid. Hempseed oil has shown success for many skin issues, including excessive dry skin, acne and psoriasis.

HOLY BASIL OIL. This essential oil cleanses and purifies the skin.

JOJOBA OIL. Technically a wax, jojoba oil is the oil that's closest to the sebum produced by the skin. It also hydrates deeply and regulates oil production, bringing balance to oily or combination skin.

KUKUI NUT OIL. Kukui nut oil contains very high levels of linoleic and alpha-linolenic, essential fatty acids. This oil is also readily absorbed into the skin, providing the essential elements for excessively dry skin to acne.

MACADAMIA NUT OIL. Macadamia nut oil is high in monounsaturated fatty acids. Like jojoba oil, it closely resembles sebum. It is easily utilized and absorbed and does not clog pores, making it work wonders for both oily and dry skin issues.

OLIVE OIL. Olive oil is full of skin-loving antioxidants, including polyphenols (a micronutrient protects skin from UV rays) and vitamin E, which is known to preserve skin's youthfulness and help reduce fine lines.

PALM OIL. Palm oil is high in beta-carotene, vitamin E, and other antioxidants. It deeply moisturizes the skin.

RICE MILK. Rice milk is made by boiling rice in water and blending it until a milk-like texture is produced. Rice milk is an excellent moisturizer that hydrates the skin and helps reduce excess oil.

ROSE HIP OIL. Rose hip oil is full of antioxidants (vitamin C) to protect your skin cells. It has a high absorbency rate, helps rehydrate skin, improve elasticity and reduce the appearance of scarring. It also contains vitamin A, which can help promote healthy levels of collagen, thereby keeping the skin firm.

SAFFLOWER OIL. This light, anti-inflammatory oil makes a great carrier oil. It's rich in oleic acid, which is good for the hair and scalp, as well as linoleic acid, which clears pores and stimulates cell renewal.

SESAME OIL. The natural acids found in sesame oil (linoleic, palmitic, and stearic) soften and moisturize skin. It contains the antioxidants vitamin E and sesamol, which are anti-inflammatory and prevent signs of aging.

SUNFLOWER OIL. Sunflower oil is rich in the anti-aging vitamins A, C, D, and E. It also has emollient properties that help the skin to retain its moisture.

ST. JOHN'S WORT OIL. St. John's wort is known for its anti-inflammatory properties as well as content of bioflavonoid. It is wonderful for calming redness and used for sensitive skin.

SOY MILK. Soy milk is rich in proteins, which means that it can help the skin produce collagen, which is vital for youthful-looking skin. It also aids in skin cell turnover by absorbing dead skin cells. Soy milk is a good choice for vegans in place of goat or cow milk when making masks.

TAMANU OIL. A known healing agent, tamanu oil has anti-inflammatory, antimicrobial, antioxidant, and antibiotic properties. It also promotes tissue healing.

YOGURT. Yogurt is rich in alpha hydroxyl acid, which acts as an exfoliator, as well as active bacterial cultures that can balance skin. It has antifungal and bacterial properties and helps cleanse and unclog pores. Plain, unsweetened yogurt is best because it doesn't contain any additives.

CLAYS & CHARCOALS

Clays and charcoals are the purifiers of a DIY skin-care regimen; they help the skin breathe by keeping pores clear and promoting enhanced blood flow. Each clay has unique properties and benefits such as grabbing oils, dirt, and toxins from pores like a magnet. Together (and alone), clays and charcoals combat the most congested pores.

ACTIVATED CHARCOAL. In the same way charcoal filters are used to absorb impurities in water that passes over it, activated charcoal is used to draw impurities from the skin. The charcoal goes deep into the pores to pull out rancid oils, dirt, and toxins so that the skin can breathe and function properly.

BENTONITE CLAY. Made from volcanic ash, bentonite clay binds with toxins and absorbs them like a sponge while releasing its beneficial minerals. It also draws excess hydrogen out of the cells, which is then replaced by oxygen. Due to this detoxifying process, it is helpful when dealing with acne or congested pores.

DEAD SEA MUD. Dead sea mud has many unique properties that make it a wonderful addition to a healthy beauty routine. It is high in minerals such as sodium, calcium, potassium, and iron, and has been used to combat psoriasis, relieve aches and pains, detox, and increase blood flow, which helps bring nutrients and oxygen to your cells, removes toxins, and improves the overall appearance of skin.

FRENCH GREEN CLAY. Known for its absorptive properties, French green clay soaks up impurities in the skin. This process increases blood flow to the skin cells, improving circulation.

KAOLIN CLAY. This white clay stimulates circulation and is gentle enough for more sensitive skin types. It's also an astringent and mild exfoliant, making it a beneficial addition to a cleanser.

PINK CLAY. A mild clay perfect for all skin types, pink clay is known to detoxify skin, improve circulation, and increase the renewal of skin cells.

SALTS, SUGARS & BUTTERS

Some of the most pampering ingredients in your beauty pantry include everyday ingredients, such as honey and salt. In this group, you'll find some of my favorite skin smoothers, hydrators, and bathtub additions.

BROWN SUGAR. A natural humectant, brown sugar pulls moisture from the surrounding environment. When used as an ingredient in exfoliating scrubs, it deposits that "borrowed" moisture into your skin. It also contains alpha hydroxyl acid, which sloughs away old skin cells and promotes the growth of new skin.

COCOA BUTTER. Cocoa butter is filled with antioxidants at a higher concentration than even blueberries and other superfoods. Because of its antioxidants and anti-inflammatory properties, cocoa butter may help tone and improve the skin's elasticity. Cocoa butter is a great emollient, meaning it makes the outer layer of skin softer and suppler. Due to its nutrient and fatty acid content, it can actually penetrate further than the top layer of the skin.

COCONUT BUTTER. Coconut butter is full of essentially fatty acids, like linoleic acid, which helps promote the growth of new skin cells. While coconut oil is a wonderful hydrator, coconut butter contains both the oil and coconut meat, making it higher in nutrients and essential fatty acids than the oil. It's readily absorbed into the skin. Coconut butter also has antifungal properties.

COCONUT SUGAR. Coconut sugar is less refined than table sugar, which means it contains a higher vitamin and mineral content than its more highly refined counterparts. It's a great exfoliator, because its glycolic acid content absorbs dead skin cells.

DATE SUGAR. Made from dates, this finely ground sugar is less processed than white sugar and is excellent in scrubs. Dates themselves are a rich source of nutrients, so not only does the sugar slough off old skin and dirt, but it also enriches your skin.

EPSOM SALT. Epsom salt has long been used in baths for its relaxing, detoxing and muscle-soothing effects. In a bath, the magnesium gets absorbed into the skin, replenishing the body's natural levels of this mineral. It regulates electrolytes in the body, which can reduce inflammation and muscle soreness.

HONEY. Honey is a humectant, which means it helps skin retain its own moisture. It's an antiseptic with healing properties, making it helpful for acne or breakouts. Honey contains amino acids (the building blocks of protein), which are known for their anti-aging abilities. It is also a rich source of enzymes, which are catalysts that speed biological processes. Because it is both an antimicrobial and antioxidant, it protects the skin from sun damage and supports the skin's ability to rejuvenate.

MAPLE SYRUP. Much like honey, pure maple syrup (not the type made with corn syrup) makes an excellent ingredient in skin-care recipes. It's packed with antioxidants that protect the skin from oxidative damage. This sap of the maple tree also contains skin-loving minerals like calcium, potassium, and zinc, as well as vitamins A and B.

MOLASSES. It contains a vast array of vitamin such as B_3, B_6; minerals like calcium, magnesium, potassium and iron; and other nutrients, which the skin is more than happy to soak up when used topically.

SEA SALT. Loaded with skin-soothing minerals, sea salts and rock salts are wonderful in baths and for exfoliation. From Dead Sea salt to Himalayan pink salt, there are many different varieties on the market. Each salt has its own mineral composition and skin benefit.

SHEA BUTTER. Shea butter contains vitamins A and E. These vitamins help maintain your skin, health, and prevent premature wrinkles and facial lines. Shea butter contains fatty acids that replace deficiencies to restore a healthy balance to the skin.

OTHER

Here's another set of DIY ingredients that don't fit neatly into any of the preceding categories, but you will come across them in several of the recipes. Each has an important role in the preparation of your homemade beauty products.

BEE POLLEN. Thanks to our friends the bees, the abundance of minerals, amino acids, proteins, enzymes, and vitamins in bee pollen—all of which promote healthy skin—is available to us. This superfood is full of antioxidants and antibiotics, which can aid in fighting skin aging and acne. The acids found in bee pollen promote cell growth and relieve inflammation.

BEER. Beer contains yeast, which is rich in B vitamins and is beneficial in treating acne-prone skin, as it slows the production of sebum. This yeast also contains minerals and other beneficial vitamins. It's a popular ingredient in hair-care products for its ability to clean and shine. Any beer will do, because it's about the yeast, not the quality or taste.

BEESWAX. The skin benefits of beeswax are as bountiful as those found in other bee by-products. Beeswax makes an excellent moisturizer and skin protectant, which is why it's often found in body butters and lip balms.

BREWER'S YEAST. Rich in protein, minerals, and B vitamins, brewer's yeast has been found to help with acne.

CASTILE SOAP. Castile soap is typically made from olive or coconut oil, and I use it in my shampoo recipes. While it's possible to make castile soap at home, going with a natural,

---

BEST PRACTICES FOR BEESWAX

Before you make products using beeswax, there are a few tips, pointers, and fixes that I want to share to make your experience successful. Beeswax seizes very easily—when you add other ingredients the mixture can harden and become lumpy, and the ingredients won't incorporate. To avoid this, use your slow cooker to ensure temperature control and/or do the following:

- Heat oils, butters, milks, or any other fluids you are adding to the beeswax so they are warm, not cold or room temperature.

- Make sure the beeswax is hot.

- When adding anything to the beeswax stir with a small whisk or spoon.

If it starts to seize, heat immediately until it liquefies.

---

store-bought formula will make it easier to make your own DIY hair products. The recipes in this book call for the liquid variety.

EGG. Egg whites and egg yolks are a powerful skin-care team in a single package. Egg whites can help tighten pores, tone, firm, and reduce oiliness, while egg yolks contain beneficial nutrients that nourish the skin, clear up acne, and increase moisture.

GLYCERIN. Its ability to pull water from air molecules makes glycerin desirable in many formulas, as it can aid in moisturizing and smoothing skin. Glycerin should always be diluted, since concentrated glycerin on its own can dry out skin.

HYDROGEN PEROXIDE. A natural antiseptic, hydrogen peroxide is commonly used to disinfect wounds and heal skin infections. It also has whitening properties, which is another reason it is sometimes found in oral hygiene products.

HYDROSOL. Hydrosols (aka floral water) are the wonderful by-product of the essential oil–making process. When the flowers and herbs are steamed to extract the oils, the distilled water that is left behind also contains the beneficial properties of the flowers and herbs. Hydrosol is a gentle, skin-friendly way to get the benefits of these flowers and herbs. The hydrosols called for in the DIY recipes include cedar, lavender, neroli, peppermint, rose, rosemary, tea tree, and witch hazel.

KOMBUCHA. Kombucha is an ancient formula dating back thousands of years. It is made with sugar, tea, certain beneficial bacteria, and yeast. It has antiseptic and antioxidant properties. It may provide acne relief, and it's even been said to treat eczema, rashes, psoriasis, warts, and fungal infections.

LECITHIN. Derived from soybeans, lecithin is a fat that deeply penetrates skin molecules, allowing its healing properties (and others in the product) to have the greatest effect. It is high in antioxidants, very moisturizing, and often serves as an emulsifier to stabilize the ingredients in a DIY product.

MAYONNAISE. Not just a sandwich spread, mayonnaise is packed with healthy skin and hair benefits. It's generally made with egg yolk, oils, and vinegar or lemon juice and the moisture provided by the eggs and oils make this spread a good hydrator for dry skin. It also contains vitamins, essential fatty acids, and protein, all of which your skin will absorb when used in a DIY beauty treatment.

MUSTARD SEED/POWDER. Mustard is antibacterial and a source of sulfur, which is antifungal. Mustard seed helps exfoliate and hydrate the skin, and can even help with acne. It's also full of antioxidants that combat aging as well as help encourage blood flow and aid in detoxing.

NUTRITIONAL YEAST. This deactivated yeast is full of skin benefits. Its high concentration of vitamin B makes it an excellent treatment for skin conditions like acne and eczema. It also improves skin elasticity and combats oxidative damage.

SPARKLING WINE. Sparkling wine contains yeast, polyphenols (antioxidants), and acids that help promote healthy collagen, slough off dead skin cells, and remove excess oils from congested pores. The type of sparkling wine you use doesn't matter; it an excellent anti-aging ingredient regardless of taste or quality.

VODKA. This traditional Russian libation is astringent and antiseptic. Beyond its astringent properties it is used as a binder and carrier in recipes.

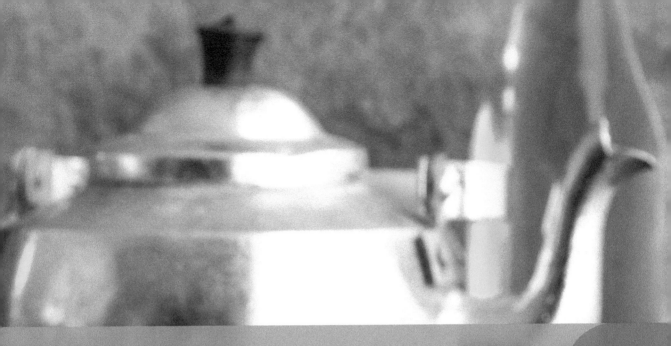

THE RECIPES

II

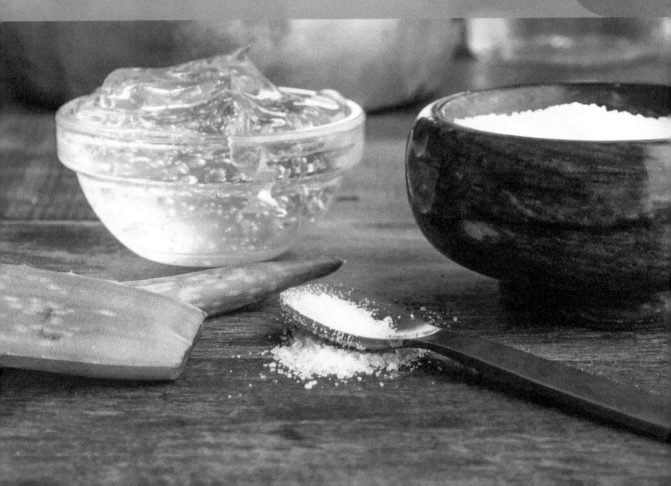

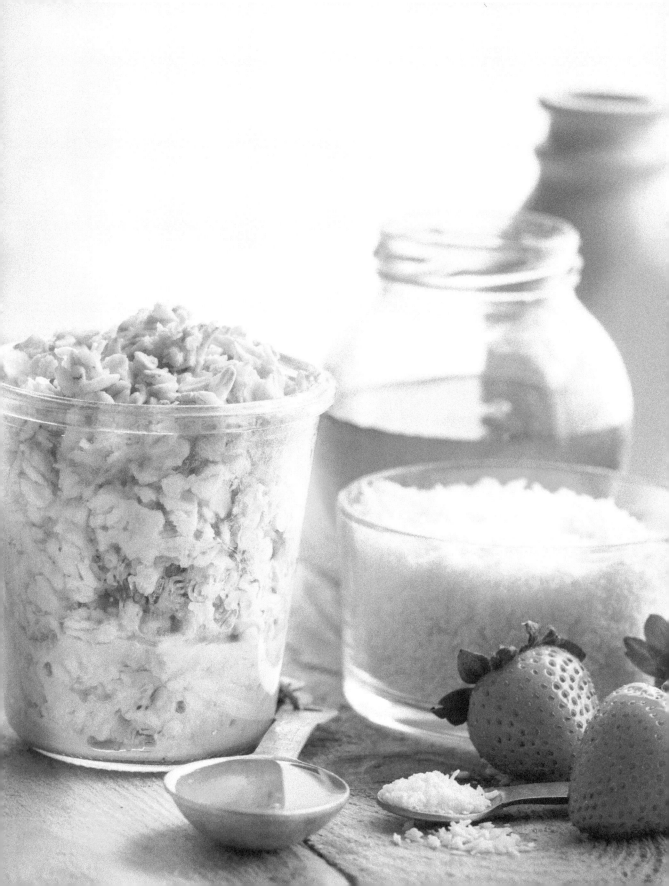

3

FRESH FACE

With everything from pollution, sun exposure, and the drying effects of air-conditioning, to the tiny bits of dirt that kick up when you walk, the skin on your face takes a daily beating. A proper skin-care routine removes chemicals, oils, dirt, and grime that have built up in pores, restores luster to tired-looking skin, preserves youthfulness, and reduces fine lines and wrinkles. In the DIY Fresh Face recipes to follow, you'll find cleansers, serums, moisturizers, masks, and facial steams tailored to every skin type that you can use daily, weekly, monthly, or yearly as needed to keep your skin healthy and glowing.

STRAWBERRY, HONEY & OAT CLEANSER

YIELD: ABOUT 4 OUNCES **TIME:** 15 MINUTES (NOT INCLUDING TIME TO COOK THE OATS)

GOOD FOR: ALL SKIN TYPES

This gentle cleanser doubles as a fabulous exfoliator for even the most sensitive skin types. The shredded coconut and strawberry seeds buff away dead skin cells, while the coconut milk and honey provide lasting hydration. This recipe is easy to make when traveling, because most of the ingredients can be found in a breakfast buffet, but in that case you'll have to use a utensil instead of your mini food processor.

1 tablespoon shredded coconut
2 strawberries
¼ cup precooked oats
1 tablespoon coconut milk (or green tea)
1 tablespoon honey (or molasses)

1. In a mini food processor, combine the shredded coconut and strawberries. Pulse a few times.

2. Add rest of the ingredients to the mini chop and pulse again until smooth.

3. Transfer to a small airtight container.

TO USE: Wash your face with a dime-size amount of cleanser. Rinse completely.

STORAGE: Store in the refrigerator for 10 days to 2 weeks. You can also make a larger batch and freeze for later use. Fill an ice cube tray with a dollop of the product in each space and thaw one cube in the refrigerator or on the countertop as needed.

USE: Daily, morning and night

A CLOSER LOOK

You will notice that the different cleansers have different textures and consistencies. Some will be a tad runnier, others firmer, and some that I call a "cleansing paste." I love cleansing pastes. They are easy to use, easy to store, and work wonders. Do remember when washing your face it should always be pre-moistened with warm water. I cannot stress enough the importance of cleansing with warm, not hot, water for proper skin health. With a paste it is even more important to make sure your skin is moistened, and you will add a few drops of water to the paste to loosen it until it spreads easily in your palms, then you can smoothly apply it to the face.

ALMOND CLEANSER

GOOD FOR: DRY SKIN, DULL SKIN

The almonds in this cleanser are rich in vitamin E and essential fatty acids, which restore moisture. By using ground almonds, not only do you receive all the beneficial properties of the almond, but also they act as a mild exfoliate.

⅛ cup licorice tea, prepared and cooled
¼ cup finely ground almonds
1 tablespoon goat milk or soymilk
½ tablespoon molasses

1. Add all ingredients to a mini chop or blender and blend well. You can use whole almonds and grind them first, then add the rest of the ingredients, and blend again.

2. Transfer to a small airtight container.

TO USE: Wash your face with a dime-size amount of cleanser. Rinse completely.

STORAGE: Store in the refrigerator for 10 days to 2 weeks. You can also make a larger batch and freeze for later use. Fill an ice cube tray with a dollop of the product in each space and thaw one cube in the refrigerator or on the countertop as needed.

USE: Daily, morning and night

ALLERGY ADJUSTMENT
If you have a nut allergy, replace the ground almonds with hemp flour.

FRESH FACE / CLEANSERS

3

ACTIVATED CHARCOAL CLEANSER

YIELD: ABOUT 4 OUNCES **TIME:** 15 MINUTES

GOOD FOR: ALL SKIN TYPES

Activated charcoal is a skin-care must for every skin type. It goes deep into your pores and pulls out all the old oils and dirt, stripping skin clean so that it can breathe again. Congested pores worsen all skin issues and accelerate skin aging. So, for deep-pore cleansing and detoxing, this is a go-to cleanser.

½ teaspoon activated charcoal
¾ teaspoon jojoba oil
1 tablespoon French green clay
2 tablespoons finely ground sunflower seeds

1. Add all ingredients to a mini chop or blender and blend well.

2. Transfer to a small airtight container.

TO USE: Wash your face with a dime-size amount of cleanser. The cleanser will be powdery or what I call a "cleansing paste," and you will need to activate it with water at the time of use. For dry masks, it takes just about ⅛–½ of a teaspoon of water for the right consistency. Rinse completely.

STORAGE: Store in the refrigerator for up to 3 weeks, or 4–8 months in the freezer.

USE: Twice daily

DID YOU KNOW?
Activated charcoal is not the same kind of charcoal we use for BBQ grilling. It's produced specifically for its medicinal purposes. Medical professionals use it to treat a variety of conditions, including poisoning. Estheticians love it for its ability to attract toxins from the skin, perhaps in the same way that it helps draw poisons from the body.

QUINOA CLEANSER

YIELD: ABOUT 4 OUNCES **TIME:** 10 MINUTES

GOOD FOR: AGING SKIN, DULL/LACKLUSTER SKIN

Quinoa feeds much-needed amino acids to your skin, which strengthen connective tissue and help maintain the skin's elasticity. Goat milk softens fine lines and wrinkles and provides the skin with a powerful boost of essential fatty acids. Pumpkin seeds, which slough off dead skin cells, are also a good source of those skin-loving essential fatty acids.

2 tablespoons + 2 teaspoons quinoa flour
2 tablespoons powdered goat milk
2 teaspoons finely ground pumpkin seeds
2 teaspoons sea salt

1. Add all ingredients to a mini chop or blender and blend well.

2. Transfer to a small airtight container.

TO USE: Wash your face with a dime-size amount of cleanser. Rinse completely.

STORAGE: Store in a cool, dry place for up to 2 weeks.

USE: Twice daily

TRY INSTEAD

If you are vegan, you can replace the goat milk with soymilk. Sometimes, the active ingredient in a recipe calls for an animal product, so there won't be a suitable alternative. In other cases, a simple switch can be made. Experiment to see what works for you.

BANANA CLEANSER

YIELD: ABOUT 4 OUNCES **TIME:** 15 MINUTES

GOOD FOR: ANTI-AGING, SKIN SOFTENING

The potassium in bananas hydrates and moisturizes dry skin. Vitamins A, B, C, and E, which are also found in bananas, protect against aging, promote the production of collagen, balance oil, and fight skin-damaging oxidation.

2 tablespoons banana flour

1 tablespoon + 1½ teaspoons powdered goat milk or soymilk

2 tablespoons lucuma powder

¼ banana, mashed (optional, for increased moisturizing)

1. Add all ingredients to a bowl and mix well. If you use the banana, blend in a mini chop or blender.

2. Transfer to a small airtight container.

TO USE: Wash your face with a dime-size amount of cleanser. Rinse completely.

STORAGE: Store in the refrigerator for up 3 weeks without banana and 10 days in refrigerator with banana.

USE: Daily, morning and night

A CLOSER LOOK

Lucuma powder comes from a fruit that is native to regions of South America. It has the consistency of a hard-boiled egg yolk and a uniquely sweet taste. High in nutrients such as iron, zinc, and vitamin B_3, lucuma powder makes a wonderful addition to beauty products. If you find yourself with extra lucuma powder, you can use it as a tasty substitute for sugar or artificial sweeteners.

COCONUT CLEANSER

YIELD: ABOUT 4 OUNCES **TIME:** 20 MINUTES

GOOD FOR: DEHYDRATED SKIN

When there is product in which all the parts have active qualities for your skin, the combination can be a powerful match. Here shredded coconut exfoliates, and the flour mixed with the essential fatty acids (EFAs) and antioxidants in the milk and meat (in the butter) makes for a fantastic coconut lovers cleanser. The EFAs help pull the dirt and grime from your skin, while the flour and shredded coconut remove the dead skin cells.

4 teaspoons shredded, unsweetened coconut
1 teaspoon coconut butter
4 teaspoons coconut milk
4 teaspoons coconut flour

1. In a mini food processor, pulse the shredded coconut until the shreds are the size of small granules.

2. On the stovetop in a small pot, melt the coconut butter over low heat.

3. Add the melted butter and the remaining ingredients to the food processor. Pulse once or twice to mix.

4. Transfer to a small airtight container.

TO USE: Wash your face with a dime-size amount of cleanser. Rinse completely.

STORAGE: Store in the refrigerator for 10 days to 2 weeks.

USE: Twice daily

DETOX CLEANSER

GOOD FOR: ELIMINATING CHEMICAL BUILDUP,
CLEANING PORES

No matter what your skin type, detoxing your skin is imperative. Keeping your pores clean and restoring your pH level are key to achieving your skin goals. Apple cider vinegar restores the skin's natural pH level and aids the removal of dead skin cells, dirt, and oils. Apples have a high malic acid content. Malic acid is an alpha hydroxyl, which brightens skin, stimulates collagen production, and removes dead skin. Lavender and rosemary hydrosols fight germs.

4 teaspoons apple juice
4 teaspoons lavender hydrosol or rosemary hydrosol
2 teaspoons apple cider vinegar
2 teaspoons honey
1 teaspoon soymilk
4 tablespoons quinoa flour

1. In a bowl or mini food processer, combine all the ingredients, and pulse or mix for about 10 seconds until blended.

2. Transfer to a small airtight container.

TO USE: Wash your face with a dime-size amount of cleanser. Rinse completely.

STORAGE: Store in the refrigerator for 10 days to 2 weeks.

USE: Daily, morning and night

TRY INSTEAD
If you don't have lavender or rosemary hydrosol on hand, you can substitute distilled water.

HONEY & CHIA SEED CLEANSER

YIELD: ABOUT 4 OUNCES TIME: 15 MINUTES NOT INCLUDING TIME TO MAKE THE TEA

GOOD FOR: ALL SKIN TYPES

This cleanser is a multitasker! Packed with essential fatty acids and amino acids, chia seeds also make an excellent exfoliator. Lemon juice provides skin-loving bioflavonoids; honey soothes, softens, repairs, and moisturizes; and rooibos tea helps balance the pH level of your skin.

1½ tablespoons rooibos tea, prepared and cooled
1 tablespoon chia seeds
4 tablespoons honey
¾ teaspoon lemon juice

1. In a small bowl, combine the tea and chia seeds. Let stand for 5 minutes.

2. Add the honey and lemon juice and mix well. If it's too thick after a few hours when the chia seeds bloom, add another teaspoon of tea.

3. Transfer to a small airtight container.

TO USE: Wash your face with a dime-size amount of cleanser. Rinse completely.

STORAGE: Store in the refrigerator for 10 days to 2 weeks.

USE: Twice daily

DID YOU KNOW?
Naturally caffeine-free, rooibos tea originated in South Africa and had been wildly popular there for decades before making its way to the rest of the world. Rooibos tea contains high levels of skin-loving vitamin C.

3

MULTI-OIL CLEANSER

YIELD: ABOUT 4 OUNCES **TIME:** 15 MINUTES

GOOD FOR: ALL SKIN TYPES

Oil naturally attracts pore-clogging oil and dirt on the skin. You will see the proof on your cotton round! Perfect for removing makeup and pulling dirt from your skin's surface, this combination of oils also restores your skin's own oil production. It has everything from vitamin C to essential fatty acids to keep skin youthful and glowing.

4 tablespoons jojoba oil
2 tablespoons sunflower oil
2 teaspoons avocado oil
1 teaspoon argan oil (optional)
1 teaspoon rose hip oil (optional)
1 teaspoon camellia oil (optional)

1. In a small bowl, combine all the ingredients and mix well.

2. Using a funnel, pour into a small airtight container.

TO USE: Moisten a cotton round with a quarter-size amount of cleanser and softly wipe over your face.

STORAGE: Store in the refrigerator for 3–5 months.

USE: Twice daily

A CLOSER LOOK

When cleansing with oils, some people like to double-cleanse and moisturize. In that case, cleanse with an oil cleanser, wash with a nonoil–based cleanser, use toner, and apply moisture.

COCOA CLEANSER

YIELD: ABOUT 4 OUNCES **TIME:** 15 MINUTES

GOOD FOR: ANTI-AGING

Cocoa powder, which is rich in anti-oxidants, has amazing anti-aging properties. The same is true for lucuma and walnuts. With the addition of goat milk powder, your skin will be both soft and protected.

1 tablespoon cocoa powder

3 tablespoons goat milk powder

2 tablespoons lucuma powder

2 tablespoons finely ground walnuts

A few drops distilled water to make a paste (for activation). Generally it will be ½ teaspoon dry mix to ⅛ teaspoon liquid to make the paste and about ½ to 1 teaspoon of dry mix for one cleansing.

1. Add all ingredients to a mini chop or blender and blend well.

2. Transfer to a small airtight container.

TO USE: After activating, wash your face with a dime-size amount of cleanser. Rinse completely.

STORAGE: Store in a cool, dark place for up to 3 weeks.

USE: Twice daily

ALLERGY ADJUSTMENT

If you have a nut allergy, you can leave the walnuts out. While they add essential fatty acids and provide mild exfoliation, you will still get some essential fatty acids from the goat milk, and the lucuma powder exfoliates.

HEMP CLEANSER

Hemp is rich in amino acids and omega-3 fatty acids. Green clay clarifies skin, cleaning it to the mid-pore, and deposits those amino acids and omega 3 fatty acids to repair and restore.

2 teaspoons lavender petals

1 tablespoon + 1 teaspoon hemp flour

1 tablespoon + 1 teaspoon French green clay

A few drops distilled water to make a paste (for activation). Generally it will be ½ teaspoon dry mix to ⅛ teaspoon liquid to make the paste and about ½ to 1 teaspoon of dry mix for one cleansing.

1. In a small bowl or mini chop, combine all the ingredients and mix well.

2. Transfer to a small airtight container.

TO USE: After activating, wash your face with a dime-size amount of cleanser. Rinse completely.

STORAGE: Store in a cool, dry place for up to 3 weeks.

USE: Twice daily

DID YOU KNOW?

While hemp is in the cannabis family, it has no mind-altering properties. When hempseed is pressed, it produces a viscous oil. While heavier than other oils, hemp oil is nongreasy and absorbs easily. It's shown success for many skin issues, including excessive dry skin, acne, and psoriasis.

SUNFLOWER & JOJOBA MAKEUP REMOVER

YIELD: ABOUT 2 OUNCES **TIME:** 15 MINUTES

GOOD FOR: ALL SKIN TYPES

Jojoba oil, which is most like our skin's natural sebum, pulls out impurities and balances oil production. The balancing of your skin's natural oil is key in keeping pores healthy. The basic rule for oil cleansers is that oil attracts dirt and adheres to it, thereby removing it from the surface of your skin. Not every oil out there will balance your skin's natural oil production, of course, but the oils included in this book are great to use as indicated. This includes the other wonderful oils in this recipe!

1 tablespoon sunflower oil
1 tablespoon jojoba oil
2 teaspoons avocado oil
2 teaspoons apricot oil

1. In a small bowl, combine all the ingredients and mix well.

2. Transfer to a small airtight container. A dropper bottle works well to keep this product in for ease of dispensing on the cotton round or to make it attractive for gifting!

TO USE: Moisten a cotton round with a quarter-size amount of cleanser and softly wipe over your face. Double-cleanse if desired.

STORAGE: Store in a cool, dry place for up to 3 months.

USE: As needed to remove makeup

DID YOU KNOW?
Sunflower oil is common for cooking but not used as much for skin care, though it should be. It is high in linoleic acid as well as oleic acid, palmitic acid, lecithin, and vitamins A, D, and E. I like to use this oil because it is easy to find and is wonderful for skin. Its suggested shelf life is 3 months, but what you don't use for cleansing, you can use for cooking.

OIL & TEA MAKEUP REMOVER PADS

YIELD: MAKES ABOUT 25 PADS **TIME:** 20 MINUTES

GOOD FOR: ALL SKIN TYPES

These easy-to-make and easy-to-use pads are perfect for travel. They work the same way as the other oil-based removers in this chapter, but the pads make them even more convenient. The addition of green or white tea provides an anti-aging boost.

1¼ teaspoons castor oil

½ teaspoon sunflower oil

¾ teaspoons jojoba oil

¾ teaspoon avocado oil

2½ tablespoons green or white tea (or a combination), cooled

25 cotton rounds

1. In a measuring cup, combine the oils, and mix well.

2. Add the tea and mix again.

3. Working in batches of five pads, dip them in the oil–tea mixture until all of the mixture is absorbed. Stir between batches to keep the tea incorporated. With such a small batch you may be able to soak them all at once depending on the size of your cup you use for soaking. If you try this, make sure to turn them, open them to see it saturated all the way through, and press them on the bottom of the cup to ensure penetration. If you do batches of five, make sure to press out any excess fluid.

4. Transfer the saturated pads to a small airtight container.

TO USE: Wipe away makeup with the cotton round. Double-cleanse, if desired.

STORAGE: Store in the refrigerator for 1–2 weeks.

USE: As needed to remove makeup

A CLOSER LOOK

The tea in this recipe gives this makeup remover an added anti-aging boost. It also drenches the pads and makes the oils easier to spread.

MINT TONER

GOOD FOR: ALL SKIN TYPES

Mint stimulates circulation, and aloe vera soothes and repairs. This toner is a perfect pick-me-up, and it's especially good for healing blemishes. However, if you struggle with rosacea, this is not the toner for you, as mint can increase redness.

FOR TEA:

1 cup distilled water
1 bag mint tea
1 teaspoon dried or fresh rosemary

FOR TONER:

½ tablespoon aloe vera juice
¼ cup witch hazel hydrosol
¼ cup of prepared tea

1. On the stovetop in a small pot, simmer the water, teabag, and rosemary until the liquid reduces by half. Strain the tea and cool.

2. In a medium bowl, add the aloe vera juice and witch hazel to ¼ cup of the mint-rosemary tea. Stir.

3. Using a funnel, transfer to an airtight container.

TO USE: Lightly moisten a cotton round and wipe over your face and neck, or spray on using a mister bottle.

STORAGE: Store in an airtight container in the refrigerator for 1–2 weeks.

USE: Twice daily

DID YOU KNOW?

Aloe comes in several forms; the recipes in this book leave a variety of them, from juice, to gel, to jelly. They are all a bit different in consistency, and if you use the wrong one, it will affect the outcome of your product—however, it will not affect the benefits of the product. If you only buy aloe in one form (juice is the most common), be aware that recipes that call for jelly will be a bit runny, but usable.

FRESH FACE / TONERS

3

CUCUMBER TONER

This cooling toner restores the skin's pH balance, kills bacteria, and removes dead skin. Cucumber helps reduce inflammation, so those who struggle with acne will especially love the calming effect.

½ cucumber, cut into thin slices
¾ cup distilled water
¼ cup apple cider vinegar

1. Place the cucumber slices in a glass jar. Add water and soak overnight. Strain and discard the cucumbers.

2. In a medium bowl, combine the apple cider vinegar and all of the cucumber water. Mix well.

3. Using a funnel, transfer to an airtight container.

TO USE: Lightly moisten a cotton round and wipe over your face and neck, or spray on using a mister bottle.

STORAGE: Store in the refrigerator 1–2 weeks.

USE: Twice daily

DID YOU KNOW?
Alcohol is a common ingredient in commercial toners and witch hazel. I often hear about people using rubbing alcohol or other alcohol in place of toner. However, this is a terrible practice because alcohol is drying, and dehydrates and ages skin. The toners you will find in this book improve skin issues safely, naturally, and effectively.

TEA TONER

GOOD FOR: MATURE SKIN

Here's a triple treat for your skin: tea is rich in antioxidants that fight oxidative damage, protect collagen, and offer anti-aging benefits. When using tea in a recipe, always stick to unflavored options, such as the plain teas recommended.

FOR TEA:

2 cups distilled water
1 bag green tea
1 bag black tea
1 bag white tea

FOR TONER:

⅛ cup apple cider vinegar
½ cup prepared tea

1. On the stovetop in a small pot, simmer the water and teabags until the liquid reduces by half. Remove the teabags and cool.

2. In a medium bowl, combine ½ cup tea and the vinegar. Mix well.

3. Using a funnel, transfer to an airtight container.

TO USE: Lightly moisten a cotton round and wipe over your face and neck, or spray on using a mister bottle.

STORAGE: Store in the refrigerator for 1–2 weeks.

USE: Twice daily

DID YOU KNOW?

Apple cider vinegar (ACV) has been one of my favorite ingredients for some time. It has numerous benefits—it helps restore the balance of the skin's pH level and restores its acid mantle (or the barrier between your skin and the world), which protects the skin and makes it less vulnerable to environmental damage, like smog, sun, and wind. ACV makes skin less prone to dehydration, and inhibits growth of bacteria and fungi. It also supplies exfoliation because the acids in ACV "digest" dead skin cells.

NEROLI TONER

YIELD: ABOUT 4 OUNCES TIME: 15 MINUTES (PLUS OVERNIGHT REFRIGERATION)

GOOD FOR: MATURE SKIN

A decadent toner, neroli works wonders for reducing redness, and the natural scent helps calm frayed nerves.

¼ cucumber, cut into thin slices
¼ cup distilled water
⅛ cup + 1 tablespoon neroli hydrosol
1 ½ tablespoons apple cider vinegar

1. Place the cucumber slices in a glass jar. Add the water and soak overnight. Strain and discard the cucumbers.

2. In a medium bowl, combine the cucumber water and the remaining ingredients. Mix well.

3. Using a funnel, transfer to an airtight container.

TO USE: Lightly moisten a cotton round and wipe over your face and neck, or spray on using a mister bottle.

STORAGE: Store in an airtight container in the refrigerator for 1–2 weeks.

USE: Twice daily

A CLOSER LOOK

Neroli hydrosol (aka neroli water) is a by-product of distilling the oil from the blossoms of the bitter orange tree. Essential oils can be caustic and should be used in small amounts and only when needed. Floral waters have the scent (aromatherapy attributes) without being caustic. Don't let these beautiful waters fool you; they are powerful skin allies. But beware all "floral waters" are not real. Read the label: If it says distilled or any other kind of water with essential oil or fragrance added, it is not a real floral water. It needs to say pure (e.g., rose, neroli...) hydrosol or distillate.

ALOE & CUCUMBER TONER

YIELD: ABOUT 4 OUNCES **TIME:** 15 MINUTES (PLUS OVERNIGHT REFRIGERATION)

GOOD FOR: ALL SKIN TYPES

This magic trio of aloe, cucumber, and witch hazel works well for all skin types. On its own, pure witch hazel does wonders for the skin, but when combined with aloe vera and cucumber, its effects are even more profound. This toner is soothing, anti-inflammatory, and anti-aging.

2 slices cucumber, cut into thin slices

3 tablespoons distilled water

¼ cup pure witch hazel hydrosol

1 tablespoon aloe juice

1. Place the cucumber slices in a glass jar. Add the water and soak overnight. Strain and discard the cucumbers.

2. In a medium bowl, combine the cucumber water and the remaining ingredients. Mix well.

3. Using a funnel, transfer to an airtight container.

TO USE: Lightly moisten a cotton round and wipe over your face and neck, or spray on using a mister bottle.

STORAGE: Store in the refrigerator for 1–2 weeks.

USE: Twice daily

A CLOSER LOOK

Aloe is not new to skin care. For centuries people have used it to treat wounds and sunburns. It can be taken internally and used on hair, nails, and of course on your face. Ancient Egyptians called it the "plant of immortality."

APPLE JUICE, SPARKLING WINE & BEER TONER

YIELD: ABOUT 4 OUNCES **TIME:** 15 MINUTES

GOOD FOR: ALL SKIN TYPES, BUT A PATCH TEST IS RECOMMENDED FOR SENSITIVE SKIN

The yeast in beer helps wipe out bacteria and slow sebum production; apple juice contains malic acid, which is known for its exfoliating properties, and sparkling wine helps restore the skin's pH level. This super trio gives this toner a resurfacing quality, helping remove dead skin and restore luster.

½ teaspoon apple juice
1 teaspoon sparkling wine
½ cup witch hazel hydrosol
1 teaspoon beer

1. In a medium bowl, combine all the ingredients and mix well.

2. Using a funnel, transfer to an airtight container.

TO USE: Lightly moisten a cotton round and wipe over your face and neck, or spray on using a mister bottle.

STORAGE: Store in the refrigerator for 1–2 weeks.

USE: Twice daily

A CLOSER LOOK

When it comes to beer and sparkling wine, neither cost nor quality affects the benefits to the skin. It is all about their active ingredients. If you buy some specifically for your DIY skin-care products, there's no need to throw out the unused portion if you don't plan to drink it. You can treat yourself with a splash or two in the bathtub, add it to a facial steam, or use it to activate the dry ingredients in a mask.

TEA & VINEGAR DETOX TONER

YIELD: ABOUT 4 OUNCES **TIME:** 10 MINUTES (NOT INCLUDING TIME TO MAKE TEA)

GOOD FOR: ALL SKIN TYPES, WONDERFUL FOR BLEMISHED SKIN

Keeping your pores clean and clear is essential to maintaining healthy skin. This particular combo of tea and vinegar is great for unclogging pores, reducing pore size, and keeping break-outs at bay.

¼ cup plus 2 tablespoons rooibos tea, prepared and cooled

⅛ cup apple cider vinegar

1. In a small bowl, combine the tea and vinegar. Mix well.

2. Using a funnel, transfer to an airtight container.

TO USE: Lightly moisten a cotton round and wipe over your face and neck, or spray on using a mister bottle.

STORAGE: Store in the refrigerator for 1–2 weeks.

USE: Twice daily

TRY INSTEAD

Depending on your individual concerns, you can make a number of substitutions to this formula. For example, in place of the rooibos tea, use chamomile tea for sensitive skin, green tea for its age-defying properties, or honeybush tea, which also fights acne.

ROSE HIP & CITRUS TONER

YIELD: ABOUT 4 OUNCES TIME: 10 MINUTES NOT INCLUDING TIME TO MAKE THE TEA

GOOD FOR: ANTI-AGING (FOR SENSITIVE SKIN, DO A PATCH TEST)

The marriage of rose hips and citrus makes for the perfect anti-aging solution. The lemon juice and rind are filled with bioflavonoids and vitamins; when paired with rose hips, they prevent aging by protecting collagen.

FOR TEA:

1 cup distilled water
4 fresh rose hips, diced, or 1 bag rose hip tea
2 teaspoons lemon rind

FOR TONER:

½ teaspoon lemon juice
½ cup prepared tea

1. On the stovetop in a small pot, simmer the water, rose hips (or rose hip teabag), and lemon rind until the liquid reduces by half. Let the tea cool and strain.

2. Add the lemon juice to ½ cup of the tea.

3. Using a funnel, transfer to an airtight container.

TO USE: Lightly moisten a cotton round and wipe over your face and neck, or spray on using a mister bottle.

STORAGE: Store in the refrigerator for 1–2 weeks.

USE: Twice daily

DID YOU KNOW?

You can give your pores a workout by alternating between warm (never hot) and cold treatments. When your pores open and close, the movement helps expel debris, oil, and chemicals in them as well as tighten and tone. To do this, freeze any of the toners in an ice cube tray. Wrap one cube in a thin washcloth. Then, while steaming or showering (or simply with a warm washcloth handy), allow the steam or warm cloth to open your pores, then close them by running the washcloth with the ice cube on your skin. Alternate a few times. Additionally, on hot days, you can use your "iced" toner wrapped in a cloth as a skin-healing, cooling treat.

CUCUMBER, LEMON & TEA TONER

YIELD: ABOUT 4 OUNCES **TIME:** 30 MINUTES (PLUS OVERNIGHT REFRIGERATION)

GOOD FOR: ALL SKIN TYPES

This recipe combines the skin-loving attributes of apple cider vinegar (which restores your skin's pH level and is rich in vitamins A, B_2, B_6, C, and E, as well as alpha hydroxy acid) with bioflavonoid-rich lemon and an inflammation-reducing tea, making it a wonderful anti-aging toner.

½ cup distilled water
1 bag chamomile, green, white, or rooibos tea
3 cucumber slices, cut thin
2 lemon slices with rind, cut thin
⅛ cup apple cider vinegar

1. On the stovetop in a small pot, boil the water. Pour the water into a large glass or mug and add the teabag. Let it steep for 10 minutes, remove the tea bag, and let completely cool.

2. Place the cucumber and lemon slices and cooled tea in a small jar with a lid. Seal the jar, and refrigerate overnight.

3. The following day, remove the cucumber and lemon slices from the tea, and add the vinegar. Close the jar and shake well.

4. Using a funnel, transfer to an airtight container.

TO USE: Lightly moisten a cotton round and wipe over your face and neck, or spray on using a mister bottle.

STORAGE: Store in the refrigerator for 1–2 weeks.

USE: Twice daily

TRY INSTEAD

If you do not like the smell of apple cider vinegar, you can use less vinegar and more tea water; however, for the full effect, use the whole ⅛ cup of vinegar.

SALICYLIC ACID TONER

YIELD: ABOUT 4 OUNCES **TIME:** 30 MINUTES

GOOD FOR: OILY OR BLEMISHED SKIN

White willow bark is a natural form of salicylic acid, which is a common ingredient in OTC acne products. This makes white willow bark the perfect natural ingredient for fighting acne. Combined with witch hazel hydrosol and apple cider vinegar, this toner reduces pimples and keeps new ones from forming.

FOR TEA:

1 cup distilled water
½ cup white willow bark

FOR TONER:

3 tablespoons pure witch hazel hydrosol
1½ tablespoons apple cider vinegar
3 tablespoons white willow tea

1. On the stovetop in a small pot, simmer the water and the white willow bark until the liquid reduces by half. Strain the tea and cool.

2. In a medium bowl, combine 3 tablespoons white willow tea and the remaining ingredients.

3. Using a funnel, transfer to an airtight container.

TO USE: Lightly moisten a cotton round and wipe over your face and neck, or spray on using a mister bottle.

STORAGE: Store in the refrigerator for 1–2 weeks.

USE: Twice daily

A CLOSER LOOK

Distilled water has been heat treated to remove impurities. That's why it's the preferred type of water to use in your DIY products. However, if you only have tap water available, that's okay too and if you can run it through a filter, even better.

ARGAN, CARROT & SESAME MOISTURIZER

YIELD: 1 OUNCE **TIME:** 15 MINUTES

GOOD FOR: ALL SKIN TYPES

This combination of easy-to-source oils is a powerful ally when it comes to restoring, mending, and healing skin. Each ingredient has great transdermal penetration for optimum results. Carrots are high in vitamin A, argan oil contains vitamin E and allows for quick absorption of essential fatty acids, while sesame oil helps protect against sun damage.

1 teaspoon argan oil
1 teaspoon safflower oil
1 teaspoon carrot oil
1 teaspoon olive oil
1 teaspoon sesame seed oil
1 teaspoon sunflower oil

1. In a small bowl, combine all the ingredients and mix well.

2. Using a funnel, transfer to an airtight container. A dropper bottle works well for ease of applying.

TO USE: With your fingertips, massage into the face and neck.

STORAGE: Store in a cool, dry place for 2–3 months, or in the refrigerator for 3–4 months.

USE: Twice daily

TRY INSTEAD

As an alternative to this multi-oil mixture, you can use straight jojoba oil. This is the oil that most closely matches the sebum our skin creates. Just a few drops are needed for maximum effectiveness in regulating your skin's oil production and maintaining healthy pores.

ST. JOHN'S WORT, HEMP & AVOCADO MOISTURIZER

YIELD: 1 OUNCE **TIME:** 15 MINUTES

GOOD FOR: ALL SKIN TYPES

This moisturizer combines the actives in hemp oil with the calming effects of St. John's wort. Meanwhile, avocado promotes collagen health, and apricot oil repairs and nourishes. While this is a great product for everyone, people with sensitive skin especially love it.

1 tablespoon St. John's wort oil

1 teaspoon avocado oil

1 teaspoon apricot oil

1 teaspoon hemp oil

1. In a small bowl, combine all the ingredients and mix well.

2. Using a funnel, transfer to an airtight container. A dropper bottle works well for ease of applying.

TO USE: With your fingertips, massage into the face and neck.

STORAGE: Store in a cool, dry place for 2–3 months, or in the refrigerator for 3–4 months.

USE: Twice daily

A CLOSER LOOK

I love hemp oil because it is rich in amino acids and essential fatty acids. However, this oil goes rancid fairly quickly, so be sure to keep its shelf life in mind when using it for your DIY products.

MACADAMIA, KUKUI NUT & AVOCADO MOISTURIZER

YIELD: ABOUT 1 OUNCE **TIME:** 15 MINUTES

GOOD FOR: DRY SKIN

Macadamia nuts are packed with palmitoleic acid, which helps delay the skin's aging process; oleic acid, which regenerates and moisturizes; and phytosterols, the building blocks of plant cell membranes. All these properties repair the skin and allow for deep penetration. Combined with the high essential fatty acid content of kukui nuts, this moisturizer is a perfect treatment for dehydrated skin.

1 tablespoon macadamia nut oil
2 teaspoons avocado oil
1 teaspoon kukui nut oil
½ teaspoon rose hip oil

1. In a small bowl, combine all the ingredients and mix well.

2. Using a funnel, transfer to an airtight container. A dropper bottle works well for ease of applying.

TO USE: With your fingertips, massage into the face and neck.

STORAGE: Store in a cool, dry place for 2–3 months, or in the refrigerator for 3–4 months.

USE: Twice daily or use as a night treatment and another moisturizer for day.

DID YOU KNOW?
Kukui nut oil has a long history of use in Hawaii, most notably as an ingredient in beauty-care products. The candlenut tree from which it is derived (specifically from the nuts) isn't actually a tree that's native to Hawaii. It was introduced to the islands by early Polynesian settlers.

AVOCADO, YOGURT & BREWER'S YEAST MASK

YIELD: ABOUT 2 OUNCES (APPROXIMATELY 3 MASK APPLICATIONS) **TIME:** 20 MINUTES

GOOD FOR: ALL SKIN TYPES

Avocado, yogurt, and brewer's yeast are an intense trio packed with benefits for all skin types. This mask can be used as often as you'd like and you will see the results glowing on your skin.

2 teaspoons mashed avocado
1 teaspoon mashed banana
4 teaspoons yogurt
¼ teaspoon brewer's yeast
2 teaspoons coconut milk

1. In a mini food processer, purée the avocado and banana.

2. Add the remaining ingredients to the food processer and pulse a few times to combine.

3. Transfer to an airtight container.

TO USE: Apply 1–2 teaspoons of the mask to your face, starting at the bottom of your neck and spreading upward, avoiding the eyes, nostrils, and lips. Leave on for 5–15 minutes. Rinse off with warm water.

STORAGE: Store in the refrigerator for up to 1 week. You can also prepare several applications and freeze in single-serving portions for up to 4–8 months.

USE: As needed

DID YOU KNOW?
Brewer's yeast has gained some popularity for those who are looking for internal wonder foods, but topically it is just as rich. The same reason it is gaining steam for eating is the benefits it has for your skin. It is a rich source of minerals (especially selenium) filled with protein (all the essential amino acids) B-complex, and vitamin C, as well as shows antibacterial properties.

BEE POLLEN, ROOIBOS & BENTONITE CLAY MASK

YIELD: ABOUT 2 OUNCES (APPROXIMATELY 3 MASK APPLICATIONS) **TIME:** 5 MINUTES

GOOD FOR: ACNE-PRONE SKIN, CONGESTED PORES

This mask is the perfect solution for clearing up breakouts. Use it at the first sign of pimples, but not as a preventive measure—consider this the medicine you use to help heal, not the vitamin you take to shore up your immune system.

1 teaspoon rooibos tea, prepared and cooled
4 teaspoons bentonite clay
¼ teaspoon activated charcoal
½ teaspoon ground bee pollen

1. In a small bowl, combine tea, the clay, charcoal, and bee pollen. Mix well. The tea can sometimes be hard to mix in the powders in such a small amount. If you have trouble, use a fine wire mesh strainer and push the mixture through it to help distribute the tea in the powder evenly.

2. Transfer to an airtight container.

TO USE: Activate the mask with water or rooibos tea. For each teaspoon of mask, use a scant ¼ teaspoon of water or rooibos tea. Apply 1–2 teaspoons of the mask to your face, starting at the bottom of your neck and spreading upward, avoiding the eyes, nostrils, and lips. Leave on for 5–15 minutes. Rinse off with warm water.

STORAGE: Store in the refrigerator for 2–3 weeks.

USE: Once or twice per week

DID YOU KNOW?
Bee pollen is rich in acne-fighting essential fatty acids, B vitamins, zinc, and antioxidants. If you struggle with acne, eat ⅛ teaspoon of bee pollen each day. You can eat it straight off the spoon or dust it on salads, toast, or cereal. You can even mix it into smoothies.

PAPRIKA, HONEY & BUTTERMILK MASK

YIELD: ABOUT 2 OUNCES (APPROXIMATELY 3 MASK APPLICATIONS) **TIME:** 15 MINUTES

GOOD FOR: MATURE SKIN

Paprika is the star of this mask! It's an amazing, multitalented ingredient that fights aging, and acne, and evens out skin tone. Paired with honey to soothe, mend, and bring moisture to the skin, as well as buttermilk for its essential fatty acids, this mask is the perfect anti-aging skin boost. If you still have youthful skin, you don't need this mask quite yet.

⅛ teaspoon paprika
2 tablespoons honey
2 tablespoons buttermilk

1. In a small bowl or mini chop, combine the paprika, honey, and buttermilk. Mix well.

2. Transfer to an airtight container.

Some people can be sensitive to paprika, so do a patch test and start with ⅛ of a teaspoon. If all goes well, you can increase the paprika to ¼ teaspoon the next time you make it. Remember to do another patch test if you increase the paprika.

TO USE: Apply 1–2 teaspoons of the mask to your face, starting at the bottom of your neck and spreading upward, avoiding the eyes, nostrils, and lips. Leave on for 5–15 minutes. Rinse off with warm water.

STORAGE: Store in the refrigerator for up to 1–2 weeks. You can also prepare several applications and freeze in single-serving portions for up to 4–8 months.

USE: One to two times per week, or as needed

DID YOU KNOW?
We hear it more and more, "eat your rainbow." I love that phrase—it reminds us to keep our diets on the right track. Each color can be loosely associated with different healing properties. The color of paprika gives us insight into its skin benefits—it's filled with beta-carotene, which converts to vitamin A. Just remember that a little goes a long way, so be careful not to overuse it.

TURMERIC, YOGURT & HONEY MASK

YIELD: ABOUT 2 OUNCES (APPROXIMATELY 3 MASK APPLICATIONS) **TIME:** 15 MINUTES

GOOD FOR: MATURE SKIN

When used properly, turmeric works wonders on the skin. It's anti-inflammatory so it's good for acne. It also, reduces wrinkles and is filled with antioxidants. But be careful: too much turmeric can temporarily turn lighter skin tones yellow. Start slowly: Test a small amount of this mask on the inside of your wrist before applying it to your face.

⅛ to ¼ teaspoon fresh or powdered turmeric
2 tablespoons plain yogurt
1 tablespoon honey
2 teaspoons rice milk

1. In a small bowl or mini chop, combine all the ingredients and mix well.

2. Transfer to an airtight container.

TO USE: Apply 1–2 teaspoons of the mask to your face, starting at the bottom of your neck and spreading upward, avoiding the eyes, nostrils, and lips. Leave on for 5–15 minutes. Rinse off with warm water.

STORAGE: Store in the refrigerator for up to 1–2 weeks. You can also prepare several applications and freeze in single-serving portions for up to 4–8 months.

USE: Twice per week

CHARCOAL, COFFEE & CLAY MASK

YIELD: ABOUT 2 OUNCES (APPROXIMATELY 3 MASK APPLICATIONS) **TIME:** 15 MINUTES

GOOD FOR: DEEP-PORE CLEANSING

This mask is a great pore detoxifier. Vinegar and coffee combined with the clay deep cleans your pores while keeping puffiness at bay. This leaves your face in tip-top shape.

4 teaspoons kaolin clay
1 teaspoon French green clay
1 teaspoon Dead Sea mud
¼ teaspoon activated charcoal

MIX IN THE FOLLOWING TO MAKE A PASTE:
⅛ teaspoon apple cider vinegar
¼ teaspoon brewed black coffee
⅛ teaspoon distilled water

1. In a small bowl, combine clays, sea mud, and charcoal, and mix well.

2. Transfer to an airtight container.

3. To activate the mask, add the apple cider vinegar and the coffee to the dry mixture and mix to a thin paste. Use ¼ teaspoon of apple cider vinegar/coffee/water mixture to 1 teaspoon dry clay mixture.

4. Set aside the remaining dry mixture for the next use.

TO USE: Apply 1–2 teaspoons of the mask to your face, starting at the bottom of your neck and spreading upward, avoiding the eyes, nostrils, and lips. Leave on for 5–15 minutes. Rinse off with warm water.

STORAGE: Clay mixture can be stored for 3–4 months in an airtight container in a cool, dry cupboard. Store activated mask in the refrigerator for up to 1–2 weeks. You can also prepare several applications of the activated mask and freeze in single-serving portions for up to 4–8 months.

USE: Once per week

GIFT IT
Package the dry ingredients in a small mason jar and tie off with a ribbon. Include instructions for activating and using the mask.

DEAD SEA MUD, KOMBUCHA & BREWER'S YEAST MASK

YIELD: ABOUT 2 OUNCES (APPROXIMATELY 3 MASK APPLICATIONS) **TIME:** 15 MINUTES

GOOD FOR: ALL SKIN TYPES

This combination of unique ingredients makes for a great pore-cleansing mask. Sea mud acts to open pores and pull out dirt, while the kombucha and yeast improve the skin's elasticity and remove dead skin, along with providing powerful antibacterial properties.

2 tablespoons Dead Sea mud

2 teaspoons arrowroot

2 teaspoons rose hydrosol

2 teaspoons brewer's yeast

4 teaspoons unflavored kombucha

½ teaspoon maple syrup

1. In a small bowl or mini chop, combine all the ingredients and mix well.

2. To balance the texture, you can add more clay (to thicken) or kombucha (to thin).

3. Transfer to an airtight container.

TO USE: Apply 1–2 teaspoons of the mask to your face, starting at the bottom of your neck and spreading upward, avoiding the eyes, nostrils, and lips. Leave on for 5–15 minutes. Rinse off with warm water.

STORAGE: Store in the refrigerator for up to 1–2 weeks. You can also prepare several applications and freeze in single-serving portions for up to 4–8 months.

USE: Once per week

TRY INSTEAD

If you do not have rose hydrosol on hand, replace it with an additional teaspoon of kombucha.

GOAT MILK, AVOCADO & HONEY MASK

GOOD FOR: DRY SKIN, MATURE SKIN

This gentle, nurturing mask protects and heals the skin with its soothing properties. It's a perfect moisture boost for when your skin is feeling dry and flakey.

1 teaspoon avocado
4 teaspoons goat milk
4 teaspoons honey

1. In a mini food processor, purée the avocado.

2. Add the goat milk and honey, and pulse a few more times.

3. Transfer to an airtight container.

TO USE: Apply 1–2 teaspoons of the mask to your face, starting at the bottom of your neck and spreading upward, avoiding the eyes, nostrils, and lips. Leave on for 5–15 minutes. Rinse off with warm water.

STORAGE: Store in the refrigerator for up to 1–2 weeks. You can also prepare several applications and freeze in single-serving portions for up to 4–8 months.

USE: As needed

DID YOU KNOW?
Fresh ingredients are best whenever possible, but if you want to save time and freeze most of the masks for later use, try tripling or quadrupling each of the ingredients.

PUMPKIN, COCONUT & BROWN SUGAR MASK

YIELD: ABOUT 2 OUNCES (APPROXIMATELY 3 MASK APPLICATIONS) **TIME:** 15 MINUTES

GOOD FOR: ALL SKIN TYPES, BUT ESPECIALLY MATURE OR DRY SKIN

Although pumpkin is a favorite on the fall dessert table, it's also great for your skin. It's filled with nutrients, including vitamin A, vitamin C, calcium, and beta-carotene. Pumpkin is also great because it draws the other nutrients deeper into your skin for more beneficial results.

2 teaspoons pumpkin purée

1 tablespoon coconut milk

½ teaspoon honey

½ teaspoon brown sugar

1 teaspoon clay (optional, for additional pore cleaning)

1. In a bowl or mini chop, combine all the ingredients and mix till smooth. If you choose to add the clay, add an additional ½ teaspoon of coconut milk.

2. Transfer to an airtight container.

TO USE: Apply 1–2 teaspoons of the mask to your face, starting at the bottom of your neck and spreading upward, avoiding the eyes, nostrils, and lips. Leave on for 5–15 minutes. Rinse off with warm water.

STORAGE: Store in the refrigerator for 1–2 weeks. You can also prepare several applications and freeze in single-serving portions for up to 4–8 months.

USE: One to two times per week

DID YOU KNOW?

Pumpkin is rich in vitamin A, which is why you see it used in many OTCs—pumpkin helps the other ingredients deeply penetrate your skin.

STRAWBERRY, CITRUS & MAPLE MASK

YIELD: ABOUT 2 OUNCES (APPROXIMATELY 3 MASK APPLICATIONS) **TIME:** 30 MINUTES

GOOD FOR: ALL SKIN TYPES, ESPECIALLY MATURE OR DRY SKIN

This delicious-smelling mask doubles as an everyday skin cleanser; you might even be attempted to eat it, but save it for your skin!

FOR TEA:

1 cup distilled water
1 teaspoon citrus rind

FOR MASK:

2 tablespoons strawberry jelly
½ teaspoon maple syrup
½ teaspoon apple juice
¼ teaspoon citrus juice
1 teaspoon of prepared citrus rind tea

1. On the stovetop in a small pot, bring the water to a boil. Remove from the heat and add the citrus rind. Steep for 15 minutes. Strain the tea and cool, reserving the citrus rind tea.

2. In a small bowl, combine the jelly, maple syrup, and apple juice, and mix well.

3. Add citrus juice and 1 teaspoon of the prepared citrus rind tea, and mix again.

4. Transfer to an airtight container.

TO USE: Apply 1–2 teaspoons of the mask to your face, starting at the bottom of your neck and spreading upward, avoiding the eyes, nostrils, and lips. Leave on for 5–15 minutes. Rinse off with warm water.

STORAGE: Store in the refrigerator for 1–2 weeks. You can also prepare several applications and freeze in single-serving portions for up to 4–8 months.

USE: As needed

A CLOSER LOOK

Alpha hydroxy acids, which are contained in citrus, may cause skin sensitivity and redness in some people. Before using, apply a small amount on your inner wrist or a dime-size amount on your cheek and do a patch test by leaving it on for 5–15 minutes to see if redness occurs. If redness occurs, try a different recipe.

SPARKLING WINE, ROSE & CLAY MASK

YIELD: 1 OUNCE (APPROXIMATELY 1–2 MASKS APPLICATIONS) **TIME:** 15 MINUTES

GOOD FOR: ALL SKIN TYPES, ESPECIALLY MATURE OR DRY SKIN

By combining the powerful anti-aging actives in roses and sparkling wine, and the cleaning and detoxing elements of clay, this mask is a wonderful mid-pore cleaning, anti-aging dream.

½ **egg white**
½ **tablespoon clay**
½ **tablespoon rose jelly**
½ **tablespoon sparkling wine**

1. In a small bowl, whisk the egg white until stiff.

2. Fold in the clay and jelly. Mix well.

3. Add the sparkling wine and mix.

4. Transfer to an airtight container.

TO USE: Apply 1–2 teaspoons of the mask to your face, starting at the bottom of your neck and spreading upward, avoiding the eyes, nostrils, and lips. Leave on for 5–15 minutes. Rinse off with warm water.

STORAGE: Store in the refrigerator for up to 1 week. Although the effects of the mask will not diminish, after the first day it will not appear as attractive. The fluff from the egg white may separate. Remix with a spoon and apply. You can also prepare several applications and freeze in single-serving portions for up to 4–8 months.

USE: As needed

TRY INSTEAD

If you don't have any rose jelly, you can replace it with honey, which still makes a great mask.

PAPAYA, PINEAPPLE & PINK CLAY MASK

YIELD: ABOUT 2 OUNCES (APPROXIMATELY 3 MASK APPLICATIONS)
TIME: 15 MINUTES NOT INCLUDING TIME TO MAKE THE TEA

GOOD FOR: ALL SKIN TYPES

When your skin gets stuck in a rut, this is the perfect mask for a quick turnaround. It is an effective, natural skin-resurfacing peel that keeps pores functioning properly.

1 tablespoon mashed papaya
½ tablespoon pineapple juice
1 tablespoon pink clay
½ teaspoon licorice tea, prepared and cooled

1. In a mini food processor, combine the papaya, juice, and clay, and pulse for 10 to 15 seconds, or until blended.

2. Add the licorice tea. Pulse for a few more seconds.

3. Transfer to an airtight container.

TO USE: Apply 1–2 teaspoons of the mask to your face, starting at the bottom of your neck and spreading upward, avoiding the eyes, nostrils, and lips. Leave on for 5–15 minutes. Rinse off with warm water.

STORAGE: Store in the refrigerator for 1–2 weeks. You can also prepare several applications and freeze in single-serving portions for up to 4–8 months.

USE: One to two times per week

DID YOU KNOW?
Papaya is a well-known, natural beauty-care ingredient with many benefits. It contains an enzyme called papain, which absorbs dead skin cells, making it the perfect addition to masks. This recipe calls for only a little papaya, so be sure to enjoy the fruit as a tasty, health-promoting dessert.

COCOA POWDER, BUTTERMILK & EGG WHITE MASK

YIELD: ABOUT 2 OUNCES (APPROXIMATELY 3 MASK APPLICATIONS) **TIME:** 15 MINUTES

GOOD FOR: AGE DEFYING

This age-defying, pore-reducing mask might just become one of your favorites. Cocoa powder has both caffeine and theobromine, which are used to tighten skin and reduce puffiness. Along with the toning and tightening properties of egg white, combined with essential fatty acids and lactic acid in buttermilk, this mask is a chocolate delight.

½ **egg white**
½ **tablespoon cocoa powder**
½ **tablespoon buttermilk**
1 **teaspoon date sugar**
1 **teaspoon yogurt**

1. In a small bowl, whisk the egg white until stiff.

2. Fold in the remaining ingredients, and mix well.

3. Transfer to an airtight container.

TO USE: Apply 1–2 teaspoons of the mask to your face, starting at the bottom of your neck and spreading upward, avoiding the eyes, nostrils, and lips. Leave on for 5–15 minutes. Rinse off with warm water.

STORAGE: Store in the refrigerator for 1–2 weeks. You can also prepare several applications and freeze in single-serving portions for up to 4–8 months.

USE: One to two times per week

TRY INSTEAD

If you don't have date sugar on hand, coconut sugar works just as well.

PINK CLAY, COCONUT MILK & ST. JOHN'S WORT MASK

YIELD: ABOUT 2 OUNCES (APPROXIMATELY 3 MASK APPLICATIONS) **TIME:** 30 MINUTES

GOOD FOR: ALL SKIN TYPES, ESPECIALLY SENSITIVE SKIN

Pink clay is considered the mildest of all clays, which makes it a wonderful choice for those with sensitive skin. Use this mask whenever your skin could benefit from a detox or to help repair skin damage. St. John's wort is a perfect remedy for that!

FOR THE TEA:

1 cup distilled water
½ cup St. John's wort flowers

FOR THE MASK:

1 tablespoon avocado
4 tablespoons pink clay
1 tablespoon coconut milk
1 tablespoon of the prepared St. John's wort tea

DID YOU KNOW?

St. John's wort day comes once a year—a day when the flower, from which the oil is derived, is at its peak for picking. One year, on a road trip with my family, there was so much St. John's wort in bloom all over the side of the road, I decided we needed to pull over and harvest (or "liberate," as my daughters like to call it) some and make our own oil. After the harvest, we spent hours picking flowers off the stalks, then infused the blossoms in organic oil. What we didn't know at the time—St. John's wort flowers dye your skin bright red; we had blood-red hands for days!

1. On the stovetop in a small pot, simmer the water, and add St. John's wort flowers. Continue to simmer until the liquid is reduced by half. Strain the tea and cool.

2. In a mini food processor, pulse the avocado a few times.

3. Add the clay, coconut milk, and 1 tablespoon of the prepared St. John's wort tea, and pulse a few more times to mix.

4. Transfer to an airtight container.

TO USE: Apply 1–2 teaspoons of the mask to your face, starting at the bottom of your neck and spreading upward, avoiding the eyes, nostrils, and lips. Leave on for 5–15 minutes. Rinse off with warm water.

STORAGE: Store in the refrigerator for 1–2 weeks. You can also prepare several applications and freeze in single-serving portions for up to 4–8 months.

USE: One to two times per week

LEMON, ORANGE, GRAPEFRUIT & LIME FACIAL STEAM

YIELD: 1 TREATMENT **TIME:** 15 MINUTES

GOOD FOR: ANTI-AGING

The bioflavonoids in the peel of citrus fruits are excellent preventive remedies for skin.

2 cups distilled water
1 teaspoon lemon peel
1 teaspoon orange peel
1 teaspoon grapefruit peel
1 teaspoon lime peel

1. On the stovetop in a small pot, heat the water until it's very hot, but not boiling.

2. Add all the ingredients to the pot and simmer for 3 minutes. Remove from the heat.

3. Use immediately.

TO USE: Pour the contents of the pot into a large bowl and allow to cool until the steam is warm. Place a towel over your head, and lower your face down until you're about 8–12 inches from the bowl. Steam for 5 minutes.

STORAGE: Steams should be used immediately. The leftover water (strained) can be stored for 1–2 weeks in the fridge, or poured into ice cube trays and stored in the freezer for 4–8 months. You can use the leftover water as a cleansing splash, an addition to bathwater with sea salt, or to activate dry mask ingredients.

USE: Once per week

CAUTION

Always allow the steam to cool off a little before steaming to avoid accidentally burning your skin with very hot vapors. Make sure you keep your head far enough from the steam so it is a warm mist, never hot.

CRANBERRY, COCONUT & MANGO FACIAL STEAM

YIELD: 1 TREATMENT TIME: 20 MINUTES

GOOD FOR: ANTI-AGING

This age-defying dream steam sends alpha hydroxy acids up into your pores, cleansing and restoring them. Using dried fruit means less waste, and the liquid from reconstituted dried fruit will keep for longer.

2 cups distilled water
1 teaspoon dried cranberry
1 piece dried apricot
1 teaspoon unsweetened, shredded coconut
½ teaspoon dried pineapple
½ teaspoon dried mango

1. On the stovetop in a small pot, heat the water until it's very hot, but not boiling.

2. Add all the ingredients to the water and simmer for 3 minutes. Remove from the heat.

3. Use immediately.

TO USE: Pour the contents of the pot into a large bowl and allow to cool until the steam is warm. Place a towel over your head, and lower your face down until you're about 8–12 inches from the bowl. Steam for 5 minutes.

STORAGE: Steams should be used immediately. The leftover water (strained) can be stored for 1–2 weeks in the fridge, or poured into ice cube trays and stored in the freezer for 4–8 months. You can use the leftover water as a cleansing splash, an addition to bathwater with sea salt, or to activate dry mask ingredients.

USE: Once per week

DID YOU KNOW?
You can mix up the dry ingredients anytime to have on hand when you're ready for your facial steam. Store your mixture in an airtight container, then simply heat up the water and prepare the steam as needed.

JUNIPER, ELDERBERRY & BAY FACIAL STEAM

YIELD: 1 TREATMENT **TIME:** 15 MINUTES

GOOD FOR: ALL SKIN TYPES

This is the perfect steam to use when you are working on deep-pore cleansing and detoxing your skin. Together they have antiseptic, antibacterial properties to help remove impurities from your pores, as well as bioflavonoids and antioxidants.

2 cups distilled water
5 juniper berries
5 elderberries
1 bay leaf
1 drop tea tree essential oil (optional)

1. On the stovetop in a small pot, heat the water until it's very hot, but not boiling.

2. Add all the ingredients to the water and simmer for 3 minutes. Remove from the heat.

3. Use immediately.

TO USE: Pour the contents of the pot into a large bowl and allow to cool until the steam is warm. Place a towel over your head, and lower your face down until you're about 8 to 12 inches from the bowl. Steam for 5 minutes.

STORAGE: Steams should be used immediately. The leftover water (strained) can be stored for 1–2 weeks in the fridge, or poured into ice cube trays and stored in the freezer for 4–8 months. You can use the leftover water as a cleansing splash, an addition to bathwater with sea salt, or to activate dry mask ingredients.

USE: Once per week

OREGANO, ROSEMARY & TURMERIC FACIAL STEAM

YIELD: 1 TREATMENT **TIME:** 20 MINUTES

GOOD FOR: ACNE, REDNESS, PATCHY SKIN, CONGESTED PORES

This good anti-inflammatory, antibacterial steam calms your skin. Try it after a stressful day, and you'll feel the tension in your face simply melt away as the steam washes all the impurities out of your pores and off your face.

2 cups distilled water

½ teaspoon oregano (either dried or fresh)

½ teaspoon rosemary (either dried or fresh)

½ inch fresh turmeric, grated (or ½ teaspoon dried turmeric)

1 bag licorice root tea

¼ inch fresh ginger, grated (or 1 teaspoon dried ginger)

1. On the stovetop in a small pot, heat the water until it's very hot, but not boiling.

2. Add all the ingredients to the water and simmer for 3 minutes. Remove from the heat.

3. Use immediately.

TO USE: Pour the contents of the pot into a large bowl and allow to cool until the steam is warm. Place a towel over your head, and lower your face down until you're about 8–12 inches from the bowl. Steam for 5 minutes.

STORAGE: Steams should be used immediately. The leftover water (strained) can be stored for 1–2 weeks in the fridge, or poured into ice cube trays and stored in the freezer for 4–8 months. You can use the leftover water as a cleansing splash, an addition to bathwater with sea salt, or to activate dry mask ingredients. Be careful to not drip any sweat into your bowl if you want to retain and repurpose the water.

USE: Once per week

DID YOU KNOW?

I love the culinary flavor oregano brings to a dish. However, it is just as delicious—in a different way—for skin and body care. Taken internally, it can be used to fight bacteria and parasites. Topically, it helps improve acne and dandruff, as it has antifungal and antiviral properties.

LAVENDER, ROSE PETALS & CHAMOMILE FACIAL STEAM

YIELD: 1 TREATMENT **TIME:** 15 MINUTES

GOOD FOR: COMBINATION SKIN

This floral-based steam smells wonderful, but more importantly, it's jam-packed with anti-aging, anti-bacterial, and calming properties, making it great for all skin types and issues. Simply breathing in the scent as you steam your face provides a dreamy escape from everyday stress.

2 cups distilled water
½ teaspoon dried calendula petals
½ teaspoon dried chamomile flowers
½ teaspoon dried comfrey leaf
½ teaspoon dried lavender petals
½ teaspoon dried rose petals
¼ teaspoon dried burdock root
¼ teaspoon dried rose hips
½ teaspoon dried elderflower

1. On the stovetop in a small pot, heat the water until it's very hot, but not boiling.

2. Add all the ingredients to the water and simmer for 3 minutes. Remove from the heat.

3. Use immediately.

TO USE: Pour the contents of the pot into a large bowl and allow to cool until the steam is warm. Place a towel over your head, and lower your face down until you're about 8–12 inches from the bowl. Steam for 5 minutes.

STORAGE: Steams should be used immediately. The leftover water (strained) can be stored for 1–2 weeks in the fridge, or poured into ice cube trays and stored in the freezer for 4–8 months. You can use the leftover water as a cleansing splash, an addition to bathwater with sea salt, or to activate dry mask ingredients.

USE: Once per week

GIFT IT
Multiply the dry ingredients in this recipe by the number of steams you wish to make, package in attractive cellophane bags, and tie off with a ribbon. Include instructions for preparing and using the facial steam. If the recipe calls for an item such as a whole "piece of dried apricot" and you want to make a large batch for storage or gifts, cut whole fruit in pieces so it will distribute better in a larger batch.

VITAMIN C SERUM

YIELD: ½ OUNCE **TIME:** 30 MINUTES

GOOD FOR: ANTI-AGING

Heal and protect your skin with this vitamin C serum. Rancid oils trapped in your skin accelerate the aging process by breaking down collagen. The combination of bioflavonoids and vitamin C in this serum pack a big antioxidant punch to prevent the oil in your skin from going rancid.

FOR THE TEA:

1 cup distilled water
1 teaspoon citrus rind

FOR THE SERUM:

½ teaspoon rose hip oil
1 teaspoon prepared citrus rind tea
1 teaspoon aloe vera jelly

1. On the stovetop in a small pot, bring the water to a boil. Remove from the heat and add the citrus rind. Steep for 15 minutes. Strain and cool.

2. In a small bowl, combine 1 teaspoon of the prepared citrus rind tea, the rose hip oil, and aloe vera jelly. Mix well.

3. Transfer to an airtight container. This serum is fluid enough that you can keep it in a dropper bottle for ease of use.

TO USE: Apply 5–10 drops of serum after cleansing skin.

STORAGE: Store in the refrigerator for up to 3 weeks.

USE: Twice daily

AGE-DEFYING SERUM

YIELD: ¾ OUNCE **TIME:** 30 MINUTES

GOOD FOR: MATURE SKIN

This combination of unique ingredients makes for a potent age-defying blend that stands up to expensive OTC products.

FOR THE TEA:

1 cup rose water

2 teaspoons dried holy basil leaf

2 teaspoons dried rose hip

2 teaspoons dried reishi mushroom

2 teaspoons dried wolfberries

2 teaspoons dried ginseng

2 teaspoons dried bilberry tea

FOR THE SERUM:

2 teaspoons aloe vera jelly

½ teaspoon glycerin

¼ teaspoon argan oil

2 teaspoons of above tea

1. On the stovetop in a small pot, combine the rose water, holy basil, rose hip, mushroom, wolfberries, ginseng, and bilberry tea. Simmer until the liquid is reduced by half. Strain the tea and cool.

2. In a small bowl, combine the aloe vera jelly, glycerin, argan oil, and 2 teaspoons of the tea. Mix well.

3. Transfer to an airtight container. A small pump works well.

TO USE: Apply 5–10 drops of serum after cleansing skin.

STORAGE: Store in the refrigerator for up to 3 weeks.

USE: Twice daily

DID YOU KNOW?

Wolfberries, also known as goji berries, have become a popular food due their high content of antioxidants and beta-carotene. In traditional Chinese medicine, wolfberries are said to aid in sleep and reduce stress. If you have any left over after mixing up this serum, eat a few to reap their additional benefits.

HYDRATING SERUM

When skin cells are dried out, the skin ages faster. It may be itchy, thin, and lackluster. This serum not only will help replenish lost fluids, but also is rich in antioxidants and has anti-inflammatory properties. Black cumin oil fights acne and is filled with vitamins A, B, and C, essential fatty acids, and amino acids. This serum will not only restore a healthy fluid balance, but also keep acne at bay and mend damaged skin.

FOR THE TEA:

1 cup distilled water
½ teaspoon dried persimmon*
½ teaspoon dried birch leaf
½ teaspoon dried alfalfa
½ teaspoon licorice tea

FOR THE SERUM:

1 teaspoon black cumin oil
1 teaspoon carrot oil
2 teaspoons aloe vera jelly
½ teaspoon of the prepared tea

* Do not use fresh persimmon. If you cannot find the dried variety, omit it from the recipe.

1. On the stovetop in a small pot, combine the water, dried persimmon, birch, alfalfa, and licorice tea. Simmer until the liquid is reduced by half. Strain the tea and cool.

2. In a small bowl, combine the remaining ingredients and a ½ teaspoon of the prepared tea. Mix well.

3. Transfer to an airtight container.

TO USE: Apply 5–10 drops of serum after cleansing skin.

STORAGE: Store in the refrigerator for up to 3 weeks.

USE: Twice daily

A CLOSER LOOK

Black cumin seed oil has been used to fight illnesses in many medical traditions, such as Chinese, Egyptian, Ayurvedic, and Greek. This powerhouse oil has yet to become common in skin care, putting you ahead of the curve. Filled with antiviral, antibacterial, and ant-inflammatory properties as well as a multitude of vitamins, minerals, and fatty acids, it is an exceptional choice for many skin ailments.

DETOX SERUM

YIELD: ½ OUNCE **TIME:** 30 MINUTES

GOOD FOR: CONGESTED PORES

Everyone needs to do a complete skin-detox regimen at least once a year. Depending on your lifestyle and how many toxins you are exposed to daily, you may need to do a complete detox once a month. This serum complements your detox for ultimate results.

FOR THE TEA:

1 cup distilled water
2 teaspoons burdock root, coarsely chopped
2 teaspoons white tea
2 teaspoons dandelion root, coarsely chopped
2 teaspoons milk thistle, coarsely chopped
2 teaspoons dried stinging nettle

FOR THE SERUM:

2 teaspoons aloe vera jelly
1 teaspoon of the tea

1. On the stovetop in a small pot, combine water, burdock root, white tea, dandelion root, milk thistle, and stinging nettle. Simmer until the liquid is reduced by half. Strain the tea and cool.

2. In a small bowl, combine 1 teaspoon of the tea and the aloe vera juice, and mix well.

3. Transfer to an airtight container.

TO USE: Apply 5–10 drops of serum after cleansing skin.

STORAGE: Store in the refrigerator for up to 3 weeks.

USE: Twice daily

COCONUT SUGAR LIP SCRUB

YIELD: ½ OUNCE **TIME:** 20 MINUTES

GOOD FOR: ALL LIPS

This formula exfoliates your lips while keeping them plump and succulent. Sugar gently sloughs away dead skin, while coconut butter and honey add a lip-loving moisture boost.

1 teaspoon coconut butter
1 teaspoon coconut sugar
1 teaspoon honey

1. On the stovetop in a small pot, melt the coconut butter over low heat. Remove from the heat.

2. Add the remaining ingredients, and mix well.

3. Transfer to an airtight container.

TO USE: Apply scrub mixture to lips and massage in a circular motion for a few minutes. Rinse thoroughly.

STORAGE: Store in the refrigerator for 3–5 weeks, or in a cool, dry place for 2–3 weeks.

USE: Twice a week

GIFT IT

To share your lip scrubs with friends, quadruple the recipe and put each serving in a cute ½-ounce airtight container and include instructions for using the scrub.

YOGURT LIP SCRUB

YIELD: ½ OUNCE **TIME:** 20 MINUTES

GOOD FOR: ALL LIPS

Almonds exfoliate and provide much-needed essential fatty acids to plump them, while yogurt calms and soothes. Shea butter is the perfect moisturizer for lips and doesn't have the drying effect you get with many OTC lip scrubs.

½ teaspoon shea butter

1 teaspoon yogurt*

1 teaspoon ground almonds

¼ teaspoon maple syrup

OPTIONAL INGREDIENTS:

Pinch ground cinnamon (plumping)

Drop peppermint oil (plumping)

Pinch ground ginger (plumping)

⅛ teaspoon sea salt (healing and cleansing)

¼ teaspoon molasses in place of syrup (mineral boost)

Use organic sugar, date or brown sugar (mineral boost; fewer chemicals)

¼ teaspoon coffee grounds (stimulating)

⅛ teaspoon ground oats (soothing)

* Any type of yogurt will work for this recipe, even flavored yogurt.

1. In a small pot, melt the shea butter over low heat. Remove from the heat.

2. Add the remaining ingredients and mix well.

3. Transfer to an airtight container.

TO USE: Apply scrub mixture to your lips and massage in a circular motion for a few minutes. Rinse thoroughly.

STORAGE: Store in the refrigerator for 3 weeks.

USE: Twice a week

COCONUT LIP BALM

YIELD: ABOUT 5 OUNCES **TIME:** 30 TO 40 MINUTES

GOOD FOR: ALL LIPS

This is my secret formula, and now I'm sharing it with you because it truly is the best lip balm you'll ever use. The coconut milk makes it sublime. Once you try it, your lips will feel the difference.

8½ teaspoons beeswax
5½ teaspoons coconut butter
5½ teaspoons castor oil
5½ teaspoons coconut oil
½ teaspoon jojoba oil
½ teaspoon avocado oil
1½ teaspoons coconut milk

1. In a mini slow cooker or double boiler that you've dedicated to beeswax products, melt the beeswax.

2. Add the remaining ingredients to the melted wax in the slow cooker except the coconut milk. With a spoon you've dedicated to beeswax products, mix well.

3. Add the coconut milk, stir again.

4. Transfer to an airtight container. The mixture will be very hot so you want to make sure the container you use will not melt. You can also pour into lip balm tubes or small tins.

TO USE: Apply generously to clean lips as you would any other lip balm.

STORAGE: Store in a tin or container for 3–6 months.

USE: As needed

DID YOU KNOW?
Beeswax products can take a bit to master, but you will get it!

APRICOT, PISTACHIO & AVOCADO LIP BALM

YIELD: ABOUT 4 OUNCES **TIME:** 30 MINUTES

GOOD FOR: ALL LIPS

The perfect basic lip balm!

8½ teaspoons beeswax
5½ teaspoons avocado oil
5½ teaspoons castor oil
5½ teaspoons pistachio oil
½ teaspoons jojoba oil
½ teaspoon apricot oil

1. In a mini slow cooker or a double boiler that you've dedicated to beeswax products, melt the beeswax.

2. Add the remaining ingredients to the melted wax. With a spoon that you've dedicated to your beeswax products, mix well.

3. Transfer to an airtight container. The mixture will be very hot—make sure the container you use will not melt. You can also pour into lip balm tubes or small tins.

TO USE: Apply generously to clean lips as you would any other lip balm.

STORAGE: Store in a tin or container for 3–6 months.

USE: As needed

GIFT IT
To share your lip balm with friends, transfer portions to ¼-ounce lip balm jars. Wrap in cellophane and tie off with ribbon. Or you can forgo the cellophane, and simply stick a small bow right on the lip balm cap.

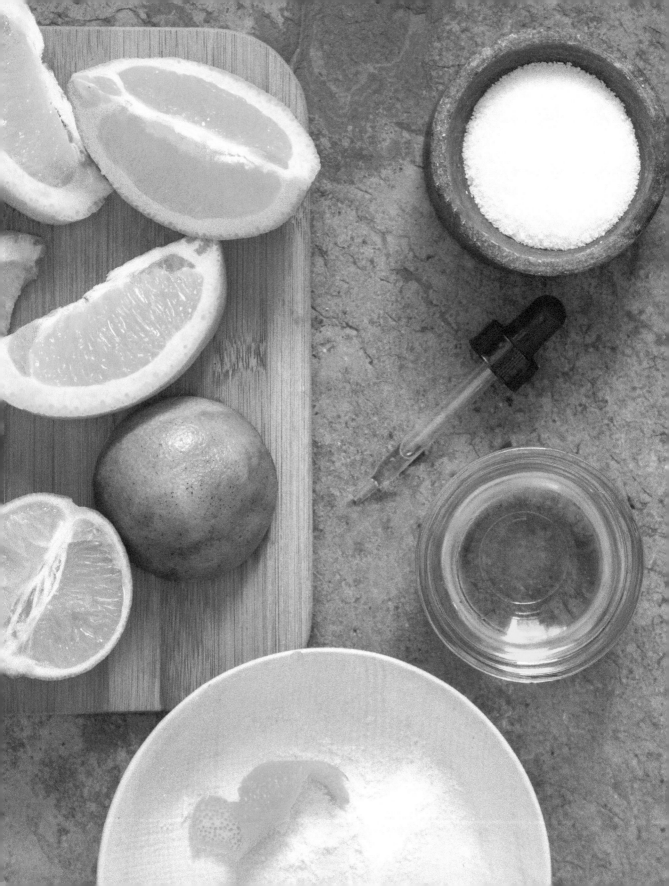

4
BEAUTIFUL BODY

B ody care often feels like a luxury we enjoy only when we have a little extra time or when it's a necessity—like bathing sore muscles, applying butters to scaly legs in the winter, or smoothing rough feet with a scrub in the summer. However, when body care is part of your daily routine, you can have luxurious skin in every season and prevent skin issues from developing. In this chapter, you'll find quick, easy recipes that bring the spa right into your bathroom and make pampering yourself simple. What's more, these nourishing scrubs, hydrating moisturizers, and molded bath bombs make excellent gifts— perfect party favors and tokens of thanks.

BASIC BODY OIL

YIELD: ABOUT 8 OUNCES **TIME:** 15 MINUTES

GOOD FOR: ALL SKIN TYPES

Many of the recipes in this chapter call for this basic body oil. This is an easy-to-make blend of some of my favorite oils. You can apply it right to your body for a dose of moisture or mix it into the recipes as called for.

¼ cup olive oil

½ cup safflower oil

⅛ cup avocado oil

⅛ cup apricot oil

2 teaspoons rose hip oil

2 teaspoons carrot oil

1. In a medium bowl, combine all the ingredients and mix well.

2. Transfer to an airtight container. A bottle with a pump or flip top works well for all the body oils.

TO USE: Apply to skin as needed.

STORAGE: Store for 4–6 months in a cool, dry place.

USE: As needed or as called for in a recipe

VANILLA-SCENTED SALT OR SUGAR

YIELD: 32 OUNCES **TIME:** 3–5 DAYS

GOOD FOR: ALL SKIN TYPES

Some of the recipes in this chapter call for vanilla-scented salt or sugar to add a natural aroma to your products. The process to prepare this delightful body product is simple.

¼ of a whole vanilla bean
4 cups sugar or salt

1. In an appropriately sized airtight container, add the quantity of salt or sugar desired.

2. Place the vanilla bean in the middle of the salt or sugar in the container and close. Set aside for a few days.

3. Remove vanilla bean from container, and set aside for cooking.

4. Reseal the container until ready to use.

TO USE: Use in recipes that call for the scented salt/sugar.

STORAGE: Store in a cool, dry place for 4–8 months.

USE: As called for in a recipe

RELAXING BATH SALTS

YIELD: ABOUT 3 CUPS (APPROXIMATELY 4–12 BATHS) **TIME:** 15 MINUTES

GOOD FOR: ALL SKIN TYPES

Made with a combination of mineral-rich salts that release muscle tension; essential oils that calm mind chatter; and avocado oil, which provides a great moisture boost—this simple bath salt recipe will provide the relief you seek.

1 teaspoon fresh turmeric or ¼ teaspoon powdered turmeric

1½ cups pure sea salt or Vanilla-Scented Salt or Sugar (page 105)

1½ cups Himalayan salt

1½ teaspoons avocado oil

1 drop marjoram essential oil

2 drops lavender essential oil

2 drops tangerine essential oil

2 drops bergamot essential oil

1 drop vanilla absolute (omit if using vanilla-infused sea salt)

1½ teaspoons lavender petals or chamomile flowers (optional)

1. In a medium bowl, combine all the ingredients, and mix well.

2. Transfer to an airtight container.

STORAGE: Store 3–6 months in a cool, dry place.

TO USE: Add ¼–¾ cup to bathwater.

USE: As desired

DID YOU KNOW?

While essential oils are typically made by distillation or expression (also called cold pressing), some plants are too fragile for this process and require a multi-step extraction method using a solvent (such as petroleum ether or ethanol) to extract the odoriferous material from the plant. This makes concentrated extract, or "concrete." The concrete is then mixed with alcohol and the final product is known as an "absolute." At the end of the process, only trace amounts of solvent remain.

DETOX BATH SALTS

YIELD: ABOUT 3 CUPS (APPROXIMATELY 4–12 BATHS) TIME: 15 MINUTES

GOOD FOR: ALL SKIN TYPES

The combination of salt, mustard, clay, and charcoal heat up your body, get your circulation going, and help draw and expel toxins from your pores. Drink a lot of water while in the bath and following it, to help the detox process. Also, be careful getting up out of the bath when you're done, as detoxing can make you lightheaded. You'll also want to scrub your tub soon after you finish the bath.

1½ cups pure sea salts
1½ cups Epsom salts
¼ cup mustard powder
¼ cup bentonite clay
¼ teaspoon activated charcoal
2 drops grapefruit essential oil
2 drops lemon essential oil

1. In a medium bowl, combine all the ingredients and mix well.

2. Transfer to an airtight container.

TO USE: Add ¼–¾ cup to bathwater.

STORAGE: Store 3–6 months in a cool, dry place.

USE: As desired

DID YOU KNOW?

Bathing in mustard powder and oil is an age-old ritual. Many spas offer mustard baths, and there are several commercially available mustard salt products. The reason for its popularity? Soaking in mustard helps open pores, encourage blood flow, expel toxins, and relieve muscle aches and pains as well as reduce fevers and cold and flu symptoms.

4

BEAUTIFUL BODY / BATH TREATS

MILK BATH

Beyond the ultimate pampering experience, this milk bath also soothes and softens. In this decadent bath, you'll be thrilled by the velvety feeling on your skin while soaking and silky skin after you are done.

1 cup powdered whole milk
¾ cup baking soda
½ cup powdered goat milk
½ cup powdered soy milk
½ cup powdered coconut milk

1. In a medium bowl, combine all the ingredients and mix well.

2. Transfer to an airtight container.

TO USE: Add ¼–¾ cup to bathwater.

STORAGE: Store 2–4 months in a cool, dry place.

USE: As needed

GIFT IT

This milk bath makes a great gift (for nonvegans, of course). A nice touch is to add a natural scent. After you've combined the powdered milks, stir in one of the essential oil blends in the book. Stir in the baking soda and transfer to a pretty jar. Provide instructions for use.

BATH VINEGAR

YIELD: 4 OUNCES **TIME:** 10 MINUTES

GOOD FOR: ALL SKIN TYPES

Vinegars might not be as popular to pour into the bath as salts are, but they're amazing skin rejuvenators. The blend of vinegar in this bath treat can soothe sunburn, detox the body, boost the immune system, ease aches and pains, help fight bacteria and fungus, and restore the skin's pH level. This combination also offers the benefits of antioxidants and malic acid (an alpha hydroxyl), helping keep the skin on your body in the same shape as the skin on your face.

¼ cup apple cider vinegar
⅛ cup rice wine vinegar
⅛ cup white wine vinegar

1. In a small bowl, combine all the ingredients, and mix well.

2. Transfer to an airtight container.

TO USE: Add the entire batch to warm bathwater.

STORAGE: Store 3–6 months in a cool, dry place.

USE: As needed

A CLOSER LOOK

Bath vinegars are versatile. You can play with this recipe in any number of ways. For dry skin, add to your bath 2 teaspoons of aloe vera juice, 2 tablespoons of coconut milk, ½ cup of prepared chamomile tea, 2 teaspoons of oats, or even a handful of chamomile flowers or rose petals (if you like floating petals in your tub). For oily skin, consider adding 1 tablespoon lavender petals, 1 tablespoon dried or fresh rosemary, or 1 tablespoon dried or fresh sage; a few citrus peels; or 1 tablespoon of clay.

ROSE, GOAT MILK & ROCK SALT SCRUB

YIELD: ABOUT 12 OUNCES **TIME:** 15 MINUTES

GOOD FOR: ALL SKIN TYPES

The clay in this scrub draws out impurities, the salt exfoliates, and the goat milk provides moisture. The rose hip is an added bonus; it's high in vitamin C, which repairs damage and protects the skin.

1 cup rock salt

½ cup Basic Body Oil (page 104)

2 tablespoons goat milk, fresh or powdered

1 tablespoon rose hip tea, prepared and cooled

2 tablespoons pink clay

¼ cup rose petals, gently ground

5 to 10 drops any essential oil (optional)

1. In a small bowl, combine all the ingredients and mix well.

2. Transfer to an airtight container.

TO USE: Cleanse your body first, then step out of the spray of the water (or turn the shower off) and apply all over your body from the neck down. It takes approximately 1 tablespoon to cover your entire body. After applying, step back under the spray of the water, rinse off, and pat dry. There is no need to re-soap.

STORAGE: Store for up to 2 weeks in refrigerator with fresh ingredients. If you leave out the tea and fresh goat milk, it will last for up to 2–4 months.

USE: 3–4 times per week

DID YOU KNOW?

Not only does the rose smell amazing, the scent also has wonderful aromatherapy properties. Rose is used to calm cranky moods. Rose hydrosol was a staple in my house when my girls were growing up. To this day, I spray it and their mood shifts immediately.

COFFEE SCRUB

GOOD FOR: REDUCING THE APPEARANCE OF CELLULITE

This scrub was popular with super-model Tyra Banks, especially after she learned that coffee is great for fighting cellulite. Used coffee grounds work best and are more effective.

1 cup used coffee grounds
½ cup **Basic Body Oil** (page 104)
½ cup rock salt or sea salt

1. In a medium bowl, combine all the ingredients and mix well.

2. Transfer to an airtight container.

TO USE: Cleanse your body first, then step out of the spray of the water (or turn the shower off) and apply all over your body from the neck down. It takes approximately 1 tablespoon to cover your entire body. After applying, step back under the spray of the water, rinse off, and pat dry. There is no need to re-soap.

STORAGE: Store in refrigerator for 2–3 weeks.

USE: 3–4 times per week

A CLOSER LOOK

If you aren't a coffee drinker, brew up a pot just for the coffee grounds so you can benefit from this scrub. There's simply no substitute for them in this recipe. You can always freeze the coffee and save it for other uses; for example, you can take a cube of frozen coffee into the shower and massage it over problem areas to help combat cellulite and fight facial inflammation.

4

BEAUTIFUL BODY / SCRUBS

COCONUT SUGAR SCRUB

YIELD: ABOUT 12 OUNCES **TIME:** 20 MINUTES

GOOD FOR: ALL SKIN TYPES

Sugar scrubs are popular because they do not sting the way salt might after shaving. Sugar is a natural form of glycolic acid, meaning that it both sloughs away and absorbs dead skin cells. The coconut combo here is sweet delight for the skin. With all the benefits that coconut has to offer—from essential fatty acids to important minerals—this scrub is a coconut lover's dream!

⅛ cup coconut butter
¼ cup Basic Body Oil (page 104)
¾ cup coconut sugar
⅛ cup unsweetened, shredded coconut
⅛ cup coconut milk, powdered or fresh
2 to 5 drops essential oil of your choosing

1. On the stovetop in a small pot, melt the coconut butter over low heat. Remove from the heat.

2. Stir the oil into the melted butter.

3. Add the remaining ingredients, and mix well.

4. Transfer to an airtight container.

TO USE: Cleanse your body first, then step out of the spray of the water (or turn the shower off) and apply all over your body from the neck down. It takes approximately 1 tablespoon to cover your entire body. After applying, step back under the spray of the water, rinse off, and pat dry. There is no need to re-soap.

STORAGE: Store for up to 2 weeks in refrigerator with fresh ingredients. If you leave out the fresh coconut milk, it will last for up to 2–4 months.

USE: 3–4 times per week

A CLOSER LOOK

To offset the naturally sweet scent of coconut, you can pair it with an essential oil like lavender or orange, or if you really like the full-on sweet, try vanilla for a yummy sweet body treat.

VANILLA, CINNAMON & SUGAR SCRUB

YIELD: 12 OUNCES **TIME:** 20 MINUTES

GOOD FOR: ALL SKIN TYPES

Even though white sugar is the least expensive and most common type of sweetener available, it contains skin-sloughing glycolic acid, so it does have sweet benefits. Meanwhile, cocoa butter adds deep moisture to this scrub, and the cinnamon and vanilla make for a pleasing scent.

1 tablespoon melted cocoa butter

1¼ cups of Vanilla-Scented Salt or Sugar (page 105)

½ cup Basic Body Oil (page 104)

½ teaspoon vanilla extract

⅛ teaspoon ground cinnamon

1. On the stovetop in a small pot, melt the cocoa butter over low heat. Remove from the heat.

2. Add the remaining ingredients, and mix well.

3. Transfer to an airtight container.

TO USE: Cleanse your body first, then step out of the spray of the water (or turn the shower off) and apply all over your body from the neck down. It takes approximately 1 tablespoon to cover your entire body. After applying, step back under the spray of the water, rinse off, and pat dry. There is no need to re-soap.

STORAGE: Store in a cool, dry place for 3–5 months.

USE: 3–4 times per week

BEAUTIFUL BODY / SCRUBS

4

CITRUS & SALT SCRUB

Basic Body Oil, sea salt, citrus, and whatever essential oils you desire make this citrus salt scrub a real skin-loving treat. The citrus peel contains bioflavonoids, which nourish your skin, while the salt sloughs away dead skin cells, and the oil moisturizes the healthy skin underneath.

1 cup sea salt
½ cup Basic Body Oil (page 104)
½ teaspoon grated citrus rind (any type)
½ teaspoon citrus juice (any type)
5 to 10 drops any citrus essential oil or a combination

1. In a medium bowl, combine all the ingredients and mix well.

2. Transfer to an airtight container.

TO USE: Cleanse your body first, then step out of the spray of the water (or turn the shower off) and apply all over your body from the neck down. It takes approximately 1 tablespoon to cover your entire body. After applying, step back under the spray of the water, rinse off, and pat dry. There is no need to re-soap.

STORAGE: Store for up to 3 weeks in refrigerator.

USE: 3–4 times per week

TRY INSTEAD
To store this scrub for up to 3–5 months, omit the fresh citrus rind and citrus juice. In place of the fresh citrus rind, use the same amount of dried rind. To dry fresh citrus rind, store in salt in an open container for 2 weeks.

HEMP MOISTURIZER

YIELD: 9 OUNCES **TIME:** 15 MINUTES

GOOD FOR: ALL SKIN TYPES

Hemp oil is wonderful for the skin. It's packed with essential fatty acids, vitamins A and E, and a host of other skin-loving elements. Hemp oil makes a wonderful daily moisturizer for all skin types and has the added benefit of keeping your skin looking youthful. The shelf life of all the oil products in the book varies, due to the fact that I take into consideration the oils you are using to make the product may themselves be old. Try to use fresh oils whenever possible so your products will last longer.

6 tablespoons hemp oil
6 tablespoons safflower oil
3 tablespoons olive oil
3 tablespoons jojoba oil
4 drops any essential oil (optional)

1. In a medium bowl, combine all the ingredients and mix well.

2. Transfer to an airtight container. Pump or flip-top bottles work well for all body oils.

TO USE: Apply onto your body where desired.

STORAGE: 3–5 months in or out of refrigerator. It will last longer in the refrigerator.

USE: As needed

AVOCADO, APRICOT & MACADAMIA MOISTURIZER

YIELD: 8 OUNCES **TIME:** 15 MINUTES

GOOD FOR: ALL SKIN TYPES

This tropical-inspired treasure is wonderful for the skin. Though it feels heavier than other oils, it absorbs easily and doesn't leave a greasy feeling.

6 tablespoons avocado oil
3 tablespoons apricot oil
3 tablespoons macadamia nut oil
4 tablespoons safflower oil

1. In a medium bowl, combine all the ingredients and mix well.

2. Transfer to an airtight container.

TO USE: Apply onto your body where desired.

STORAGE: 3–5 months in or out of refrigerator. It will last longer in the refrigerator.

USE: As needed

ALLERGY ADJUSTMENT

If you have a nut allergy, use olive oil instead of macadamia nut oil.

GOAT MILK BODY BUTTER

YIELD: 4 OUNCES **TIME:** 20 MINUTES

GOOD FOR: ALL SKIN TYPES

This body butter is easy to use and travels well. It provides your skin with long-lasting moisture. The goat milk makes your skin feel smooth, soft, and silky, while the essential fatty acids boost its moisture content.

2 tablespoons beeswax

2 tablespoons apricot oil

1 tablespoon castor oil

2 tablespoons avocado oil

1 tablespoon goat milk

1. In a mini slow cooker or double boiler that you've dedicated to beeswax products, melt the beeswax.

2. Once the beeswax is melted, add everything except the goat milk. Stir with a spoon or mini whisk that you've dedicated to beeswax products. When the oils and beeswax are completely incorporated and melted, turn the heat off, add the goat milk, and stir. Remember to add goat milk that's been warmed. See page 45 for more about beeswax.

3. Transfer to a low-profile jar for ease of use. Be mindful that the product will be hot, so make sure you pour it into a container that can withstand the heat. Silicone molds work perfectly. Use a mold capacity that will work well for you to hold and apply. I like disc shapes for body butters.

TO USE: Apply onto your body where desired.

STORAGE: Store in a cool, dry place for 4–8 months.

USE: As needed

DID YOU KNOW?

Low-profile jars are ideal for storing your body butters. The wider mouth and shorter stature make it easier to get the product out. If you use a mold, the butter will be loose so you can hold it and apply it directly on your skin for ease of application. After use, you can replace the molded butter into a container for storage.

COCONUT BODY BUTTER

YIELD: ABOUT 4 OUNCES **TIME:** 30 MINUTES

GOOD FOR: ALL SKIN TYPES

Coconut is a multitasking skin-care ingredient. That's why you'll often see it included in skin-care products. This body butter has both the active properties of the coconut's milk and meat, giving it everything from a rounded essential fatty acid profile to antibacterial and antifungal properties. It's great for the whole body, but it's an especially wonderful treat for your feet!

2 tablespoons beeswax
2 tablespoons coconut oil
1 tablespoon castor oil
2 tablespoons coconut butter
1½ tablespoons coconut milk

1. In a mini slow cooker or double boiler that you've dedicated to beeswax products, melt the beeswax.

2. Once the beeswax is melted, add everything except the coconut milk. Stir with a spoon or mini whisk that you've dedicated to beeswax products. When the oils and beeswax are completely incorporated and melted, turn the heat off, add the coconut milk, and stir. Remember to add the coconut milk that's been is warmed.

3. Transfer to a low-profile jar for ease of use. Be mindful that the product will be hot, so make sure you pour it into a container that can withstand the heat. Silicone molds work perfectly. Use a mold capacity that will work well for you to hold and apply. I like disc shapes for body butters.

TO USE: Apply onto your body where desired.

STORAGE: Store in a cool, dry place for 3–5 months.

USE: As needed

GIFT IT
For a really special treat, create a coconut-themed gift basket. Stock up on your coconut products to make Coconut Sugar Lip Scrub (page 98), Coconut Lip Balm (page 100), and this Coconut Body Butter. Don't forget your decorative jars and labels!

BUTTER BALM

YIELD: ABOUT 5 OUNCES **TIME:** 30 MINUTES

GOOD FOR: ALL SKIN TYPES

This is a true butter balm. It uses three types of butter, instead of oils mixed with stearic acid (such as "avocado butter" or "olive butter"), to make a butter-like consistency. This recipe is great for extremely dry, cracked skin, so it's a great go-to for those who live in places with harsh winters.

¼ cup cocoa butter

¼ cup shea butter

1 teaspoon coconut butter

2 tablespoons avocado oil

2 drops any essential oil or a combination (optional)

1. On the stovetop in a small pot, melt the cocoa butter over low heat.

2. Add coconut butter to the pot and melt on low heat.

3. Remove from the heat and add the shea butter to the melted cocoa and coconut butters. The heat from the butters should be enough to melt them. If not, return to the lowest setting on the stovetop and stir until melted. Remove from the heat.

4. Add the avocado oil and essential oils, if using, and mix well.

5. Transfer to a low-profile jar for ease of use and place in the freezer immediately till completely cooled.

TO USE: Apply onto your body wherever you desire.

STORAGE: Store in a cool, dry place for 3–5 months.

USE: As often as needed

A CLOSER LOOK

When shea butter melts and reconstitutes slowly, it will crystallize, or ball up. To avoid this, make sure you carefully, and slowly, melt the butter over low heat and immediately transfer it to the freezer after mixing in all the other ingredients. This rapid cooling gives you a luscious finished product.

WHIPPED SHEA & BODY OIL BUTTER

YIELD: ABOUT 4 OUNCES **TIME:** 20 MINUTES

GOOD FOR: ALL SKIN TYPES

Pure shea butter is second to none. I like to whip it to make it fluffier, lighter, and easier to apply.

½ cup unrefined shea butter

⅛ cup Basic Body Oil (page 104)

5 drops any essential oil or combination (optional)

1. With a hand mixer, beat shea butter on high for 30 seconds. To make the best whipped butter, warm the shea up with your hands (do *not* heat it). You can take the ½ cup of butter, put it in plastic wrap, and hold it in your closed hands to warm, or with sanitized hands you can hold it till it warms up.

2. Slowly pour in the Basic Body Oil and essential oils, if using, and continue mixing for 5 minutes until whipped.

3. Transfer to a low-profile jar for ease of use.

TO USE: Apply onto body where desired.

STORAGE: Store in a cool, dry place for 3–5 months.

USE: As often as needed

A CLOSER LOOK

Many OTC butters aren't made of butter at all. Instead, oils (like olive or avocado oil) or juices (like aloe vera juice) are mixed with stearic acid, which is an emulsifier, to create a substance that resembles butter. Products made with stearic acid aren't necessarily bad for you, but they are *not* real butters and will not offer the same benefits. Oils and butters have different uses and different properties. When you use the right ingredients in the right places, you'll notice a significant change in your skin while saving money by not buying those imitation butters, which are much more costly than the oil or juice they are made from and offer no additional benefits.

LAVENDER, OAT & ROSEMARY BATH BOMB

YIELD: MAKES 2 BATH BOMBS TIME: 20 MINUTES (PLUS DRYING TIME)

Bath bombs are great substitutes for bubble bath, and they go one step further: they help soften the skin as well. The lavender and rosemary in this bath bomb are relaxing and antibacterial while the oats soothe and calm your skin. If 2 bombs seem too big, you can make 3–4 smaller ones if you have the right-sized molds. See page 25 for bath bomb making tips.

1 cup baking soda
½ cup citric acid
½ tablespoon oat flour
¼ teaspoon lavender petals
⅛ teaspoon rosemary (chopped)
4 drops of essential oils, if desired
Small amount of vodka in a spray bottle

1. In a medium glass or metal bowl, combine all the ingredients, except the vodka, and mix well.

2. Spray a small amount of vodka into the bowl while mixing with your hand.

3. When the mixture begins to form, stop spraying vodka.

4. Press mixture firmly into the bottom of a silicone or plastic mold and allow it to dry overnight.

5. The following day, turn the bombs out of the mold and transfer to an airtight container.

TO USE: Place 1 bath bomb in bathwater.

STORAGE: Keep bath bombs in a sealed container so they will not lose their scent.

USE: As needed to relax

COCONUT BOMB

YIELD: MAKES 2 BATH BOMBS **TIME:** 20 MINUTES (PLUS DRYING TIME)

GOOD FOR: DRY SKIN

Both the coconut butter and milk in this bomb make it a perfect choice for replenishing dry skin. Combine all the benefits of coconut with some time simply spent soaking in the tub, and not only will your skin feel silky smooth, but you'll also feel "smooth" and relaxed on the inside.

1 cup baking soda
½ cup citric acid
1 teaspoon coconut butter
½ tablespoon coconut milk
4 drops of essential oils, if desired
Small amount of vodka in a spray bottle

1. In a medium glass or metal bowl, combine the baking soda and citric acid, and mix well.

2. On the stovetop in a small pot, melt the coconut butter over low heat. Remove from the heat.

3. Add the coconut milk melted butter, and essential oils, if using, to the dry ingredients, and mix well.

4. Spray a tiny amount of vodka into the bowl while mixing with your hand.

5. When the mixture begins to form, stop spraying vodka.

6. Press the mixture firmly into the bottom of a silicone or plastic mold and allow it to dry overnight.

7. The following day, turn the bombs out of the mold and transfer to an airtight container.

TO USE: Place 1 bath bomb in bathwater.

STORAGE: Keep bath bombs in a sealed container so they will not lose their scent.

USE: As needed to relax

DID YOU KNOW?
Putting the vodka in a spray bottle, instead of pouring it directly into the mixture, helps diffuse the vodka and produces a bomb with just the right amount of fizz. Adding too much vodka will reduce the fizz and your molded bomb will probably have a lot of air bubbles.

CHOCOLATE BOMB

YIELD: MAKES 2 BATH BOMBS **TIME:** 20 MINUTES (PLUS DRYING TIME)

GOOD FOR: ANTI-AGING OR JUST FOR FUN

The antioxidants in this bomb make it a great anti-aging soak. The combination of the cocoa powder and butter are a perfect match, because they each increase the other's potency and make this a more powerful soak. Not interested in anti-aging treatments? That's okay. This makes for a great just-for-fun bath! Kids love it, too. Make sure to help little ones out of the tub when the bath is all done, since the bomb may make the tub slippery.

1 cup baking soda
½ cup citric acid
1 teaspoon cocoa butter
½ tablespoon cocoa powder
1 teaspoon safflower oil
4 drops of essential oils, if desired
Small amount of vodka in a spray bottle

1. In a medium glass or metal bowl, combine baking soda and citric acid, and mix well.

2. On the stovetop in a small pot, melt the cocoa butter over low heat. Remove from the heat.

3. Add the cocoa powder, safflower oil, melted butter, and essential oils, if using, to the baking soda–citric acid mixture, and mix well.

4. Spray a tiny amount of vodka into the bowl while mixing with your hand.

5. When the mixture begins to form, stop spraying vodka.

6. Press the mixture firmly into the bottom of a silicone or plastic mold and allow it to dry overnight.

7. The following day, turn the bombs out of the mold and transfer to an airtight container.

TO USE: Place 1 bath bomb in bathwater.

STORAGE: Keep bath bombs in a sealed container so they will not lose their scent.

USE: As needed to relax

A CLOSER LOOK

Whenever using butters, oils, or moisturizers in the tub or shower, be careful getting out. These ingredients can make surfaces slippery. I suggest keeping baking soda near your shower or bath and sprinkling a little around before you get out.

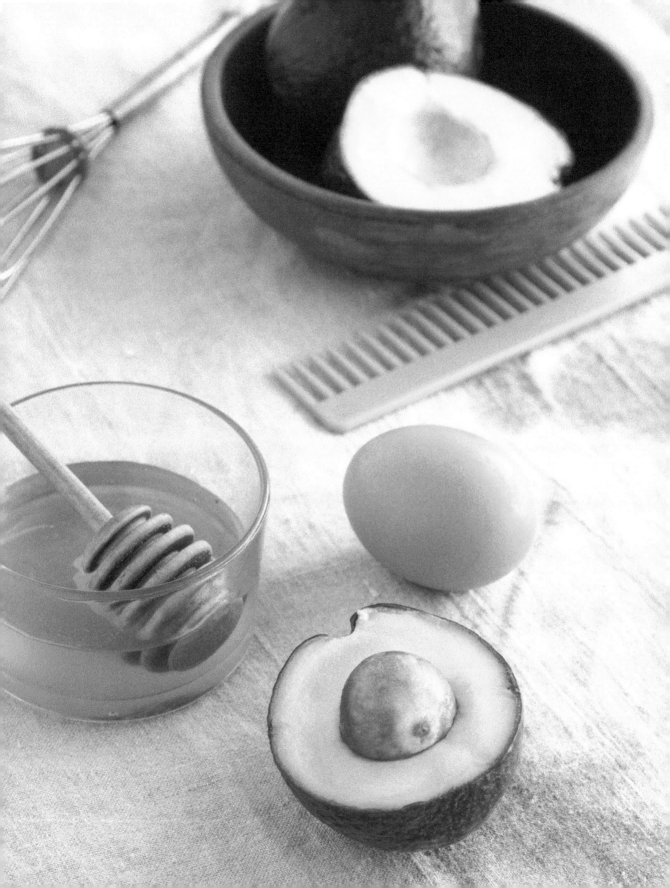

5

LUSCIOUS LOCKS

K eeping your scalp stimulated and free of buildup can promote hair growth while reducing flyaways, excess oil, and frizz. The right shampoos, conditioners, and masks can improve the quality of your mane, without artificial scents and the chemicals that create a thick lather. Do note the shampoos and conditioners feel different than the ones you buy in the store. Some shampoos do not lather and some leave your hair feeling squeaky clean. Without all the "cone" chemicals (silicone, dimethicone), these hair formulas do not have "slip"—that slick, slippery feel you may be used to—and your hair may feel a bit rough in the shower. But wait for the beautiful results!

HAIR TEA

YIELD: ABOUT 12 OUNCES TIME: 30 MINUTES

GOOD FOR: ALL HAIR TYPES

This Hair Tea is the building block of many of the recipes in this chapter. It's a nutrient-filled blend of herbs, which can strengthen and repair your hair.

3 cups distilled water
1 teaspoon dried horsetail
1 teaspoon cut oat straw
1 teaspoon dried lavender petals
1 teaspoon dried nettle
1 teaspoon dried rosemary
1 teaspoon green tea leaves
1 teaspoon white tea leaves

1. On the stovetop in a small pot, bring water to a simmer. Add all the ingredients and continue to simmer until the liquid is reduced by half. Strain the tea and cool.

2. Using a funnel, transfer to an airtight container.

TO USE: Add to recipes when Hair Tea is called for, or you can use as a hair rinse.

STORAGE: Store in an airtight container in the refrigerator for up 1–2 weeks. Freeze any unused portions in ice cube trays for later use.

USE: As called for in recipes

A CLOSER LOOK

When buying dried herbs, look at the shelf life of each one and buy them in bulk accordingly. If you have friends who also enjoy making their own skin-care products, buy the herbs in bulk and divide it among you; the more you buy, often the cheaper it will be.

COCONUT MILK SHAMPOO

YIELD: 6 OUNCES **TIME:** 20 MINUTES

GOOD FOR: ALL HAIR TYPES

One important aspect for maintaining healthy hair is to moisturize. Since hair is dead it often gets brittle and breaks. This coconut milk shampoo is filled with essential fatty acids, making it an ideal shampoo, at once cleansing and hydrating.

¼ teaspoon coconut butter
½ cup liquid castile soap
⅛ cup plus 1 tablespoon coconut milk
⅛ cup Hair Tea (page 126)

1. On the stovetop in a small pot, melt the coconut butter over low heat. Remove from the heat.

2. Put the soap, coconut milk, Hair Tea, and the melted coconut butter in a blender and blend for 15–45 seconds.

3. Using a funnel, transfer to a shower-safe airtight container.

TO USE: Shake well. Work into your scalp while in the shower.

STORAGE: Store in the refrigerator for up to 1–2 weeks.

USE: As needed

DID YOU KNOW?
To add fragrance to your shampoo, use a scented castile soap in this recipe. Dr. Bonnor's products are a good choice for this because they're pure quality and generally easy to find on store shelves.

5

LUSCIOUS LOCKS / SHAMPOOS

ARGAN OIL SHAMPOO

YIELD: 8 OUNCES **TIME:** 20 MINUTES

GOOD FOR: ALL HAIR TYPES

Native to Morocco, argan oil promotes shine and softness in hair. Called "liquid gold" by some, this oil is a natural moisturizer that's found in many OTC hair-care products.

½ cup liquid castile soap

6 tablespoons Hair Tea (page 126)

¼ teaspoon argan oil

½ tablespoon baking soda, optional for deep cleaning

1. In a blender, combine all the ingredients and blend for 15 to 45 seconds. You can mix by hand if you do not have a blender, but a blender will always give you a better finished product.

2. Using a funnel, transfer to a shower-safe airtight container.

TO USE: Shake well. Work into your scalp while in the shower, rinse, and repeat.

STORAGE: Store in the refrigerator for 1–2 weeks.

USE: As often as needed

A CLOSER LOOK

Baking soda is a highly alkaline substance, which opens the outer layer of your hair (the cuticle) and allows moisture to penetrate deeply, making it a great cleanser. However, anytime you use a highly alkaline product, the pH level needs to be rebalanced to close the cuticle shaft. The Hair Mask recipes (pages 141–147) are perfect for this.

APPLE CIDER VINEGAR & GLYCERIN SHAMPOO

YIELD: ABOUT 5 OUNCES **TIME:** 20 MINUTES

GOOD FOR: ALL HAIR TYPES

Aloe vera balances your scalp's pH level and promotes hair growth while reducing itching, inflammation, and dandruff. It also breaks down the old sebum (oil) on your scalp and removes dead skin cells for an advanced cleaning treatment. Meanwhile, glycerin is a humectant, meaning that it will help pull moisture into your hair, which you know your hair will love!

2 tablespoons baking soda (for deep cleaning) or ¼ cup castile soap (for maintenance)

½ cup Hair Tea (page 126)

2 teaspoons glycerin

2 teaspoons apple cider vinegar

1. In a blender, combine all the ingredients and blend for 15–45 seconds. You can mix by hand if you do not have a blender, but a blender will always give you a better finished product.

2. Using a funnel, transfer to a shower-safe airtight container.

TO USE: Shake well. Work into your scalp while in the shower, rinse, and repeat.

STORAGE: Store in the refrigerator for 1–2 weeks.

USE: As needed

TRY INSTEAD

If you don't have glycerin handy in your pantry, use 1 teaspoon of honey, which also functions as a humectant. Melt the honey in warmed Hair Tea so it distributes evenly in the product.

ALOE & PALM SHAMPOO

YIELD: 6 OUNCES **TIME:** 15 MINUTES

GOOD FOR: ALL HAIR TYPES

Palm oil does wonders for your locks. It keeps hair soft and elastic, preventing brittleness and breakage; it also works to smooth the hair shaft. There are two types of palm oil available—red and regular. Red is popular as it has a higher beta-carotene content, but either will work fine. An important note: do *not* use red palm oil if your hair is very blond or bleached—you may end up with an unintentional dye job!

⅛ cup Hair Tea (page 126)
6 tablespoons liquid castile soap
⅛ cup aloe vera gel
1 teaspoon glycerin
⅛ teaspoon palm oil

1. In a small pot on the stovetop or in the microwave, melt the palm oil.

2. Add all the ingredients (including the melted butter) in a blender and blend for 15–45 seconds.

3. Using a funnel, transfer to a shower-safe airtight container.

TO USE: Shake well. Work into your scalp while in the shower.

STORAGE: Store in the refrigerator for 1–2 weeks.

USE: As needed

TRY INSTEAD
Switch things up and replace the palm oil with coconut oil.

APPLE CIDER VINEGAR SHAMPOO

YIELD: 8 OUNCES **TIME:** 15 MINUTES

GOOD FOR: ALL HAIR TYPES

Apple cider vinegar helps control dandruff, and it has antifungal properties. This ingredient leaves your hair feeling squeaky clean, and don't worry about your hair smelling like vinegar; the smell fades once you've rinsed it out.

½ cup castile soap
¼ cup apple cider vinegar
¼ cup Hair Tea (page 126)

1. In a blender, combine all the ingredients and blend for 15–45 seconds. You can mix by hand if you do not have a blender, but a blender will always give you a better finished product.

2. Using a funnel, transfer to a shower-safe airtight container.

TO USE: Shake well. Work into your scalp while in the shower

STORAGE: Store in the refrigerator for 1–2 weeks.

USE: As needed

DID YOU KNOW?
Sodium laurel sulfate is an ingredient found in many OTC products that provides the rich lather we all associate with getting our hair clean. There's a debate about its safety, though, so why put it on your body if you don't have to? DIY shampoos provide the same level of clean without the question of what's safe and what's not, although with some you'll have to do without the chemical lather.

5

LUSCIOUS LOCKS / SHAMPOOS

HYDRATING CONDITIONER

YIELD: 7 OUNCES **TIME:** 30 MINUTES

GOOD FOR: ALL HAIR TYPES

During a power outage, I wanted to make quick use of the perishable items in our fridge, so I mixed up a quick and easy version of this conditioner. My daughters and their friends really enjoyed mixing up the ingredients and applying it to their hair . . . unfortunately, when the power goes out here, so does the well! When we finally found a neighbor who had access to water, everyone loved their moisturized, shiny hair.

1 egg white
1 teaspoon palm oil
½ cup yogurt, plain
⅛ cup mayonnaise
½ teaspoon glycerin
1 teaspoon aloe vera gel

1. In a small bowl, whisk the egg white until stiff. Set aside.

2. In a small pot, melt the palm oil over low heat. Remove from the heat.

3. Add the yogurt, mayonnaise, and glycerin to the melted palm oil, and mix well. You can also mix in a blender for better results.

4. When the mixture is at room temperature, slowly fold in the egg white.

5. Transfer the mixture to a shower-proof airtight container.

TO USE: After shampooing, apply to your hair (with a wide-tooth comb if you choose). The length of your hair will depend on how much you use. Rinse out.

STORAGE: Store in the refrigerator for 1–2 weeks and take only what you need into the shower.

USE: As needed

TRY INSTEAD
If you're vegan, try using vegan mayonnaise and soy yogurt.

COCONUT CONDITIONER

YIELD: 6 OUNCES **TIME:** 20 MINUTES

GOOD FOR: ALL HAIR TYPES

This triple wallop of coconut is moisturizing and nourishing, and smells delicious. For the coconut yogurt in this recipe, seek out one that's actually made with coconut milk rather than coconut-flavored dairy yogurt.

¼ teaspoon coconut butter
½ teaspoon palm oil
¼ cup coconut yogurt
½ cup coconut milk

1. On the stovetop in a small pot, melt the coconut butter and palm oil over low heat. Remove from the heat.

2. In a mini food processor or blender, combine the coconut yogurt and coconut milk. Add the melted butter-oil mixture. Blend mixture until smooth.

3. Transfer to a shower-safe container.

TO USE: After shampooing, apply to your hair (with a wide-tooth comb if you choose). How much you will use depends on the length of your hair. Rinse out.

STORAGE: Store in the refrigerator for 1–2 weeks and take only what you need into the shower.

USE: As needed

DID YOU KNOW?

Most OTC coconut conditioners have little or no coconut in them; they usually contain the fragrance, which doesn't do anything for your hair but make it smell good, or they have just a small amount of coconut that's not enough to make a difference. By making your own coconut conditioner, you know that you are using real coconut and exactly how much is in your bottle.

EGG & AVOCADO CONDITIONER

Egg yolk, avocado, and a blend of oils give this mask-like conditioner a creamy richness. I love the addition of goat milk in this recipe, but feel free to swap it out with whatever type of milk you have on hand.

⅛ avocado
½ cup Hair Tea (page 126)
½ egg yolk
½ tablespoon goat milk
¼ teaspoon coconut oil
¼ teaspoon olive oil

1. In a mini food processor or blender, blend the avocado for 10 to 20 seconds, or until smooth.

2. Add the remaining ingredients, and blend again until smooth.

3. Transfer to a shower-safe airtight container.

TO USE: After shampooing, apply to your hair (with a wide-tooth comb if you choose). How much you will use depends on the length of your hair. Rinse out.

STORAGE: Store in the refrigerator for 1–2 weeks and take only what you need into the shower.

USE: As needed

A CLOSER LOOK

Egg yolk contains a number of hair-nourishing ingredients, including protein, sulfur, and vitamins A, D, and E. When applied to your hair as part of a conditioner, these nutrients have a chance to penetrate deeply, both strengthening and softening your hair.

5

LUSCIOUS LOCKS / CONDITIONERS

HONEY CONDITIONER

YIELD: ABOUT 8 OUNCES **TIME:** 30 MINUTES

GOOD FOR: ALL HAIR TYPES

We often think of honey as a sweet treat, and when it comes to skin and hair care, this is still true. Honey is a versatile and wonderful beauty pantry staple. Filled with enzymes (catalysts that speed biochemical processes), nutrients, antioxidants, and antibacterial properties, honey also helps skin and hair retain moisture.

1 teaspoon palm oil
1 tablespoon honey
1 cup Hair Tea (page 126)
1 tablespoon glycerin

1. On the stovetop in a small pot, melt the palm oil over low heat. Remove from the heat.

2. In a mini food processor or blender, combine with the remaining ingredients, and blend for 10 to 20 seconds, or until the mixture is smooth.

3. Add the melted palm oil, and blend again for 10 to 20 seconds.

4. Transfer to a shower-safe airtight container.

TO USE: After shampooing, apply to your hair (with a wide-tooth comb if you choose). How much you will use depends on the length of your hair. Rinse out.

STORAGE: Store in the refrigerator for 1–2 weeks and take only what you need into the shower.

USE: As needed

DID YOU KNOW

Raw honey is the best type of honey to use for your skin and hair treatments. Raw honey is neither heat treated nor pasteurized, so none of its nutrient content is affected. What you get is a product with more active enzymes, antioxidants, and nutrients to benefit your hair.

MOISTURE & SHINE SPRAY

YIELD: ABOUT 2 OUNCES **TIME:** 30 MINUTES

GOOD FOR: ALL HAIR TYPES

Hair sprays are for more than just styling and holding. In the same way serums can be problem-solvers for your skin, all of the DIY hair sprays help with hair issues. This spray is perfect if you're struggling with dryness or lack-luster tresses.

½ tablespoon palm oil
½ tablespoon coconut butter
1 tablespoon vodka
1 tablespoon glycerin
½ tablespoon camellia oil
1 teaspoon argan oil

1. On the stovetop in a small pot, melt the palm oil and coconut butter over low heat. Remove from the heat.

2. In a mini food processor, combine the melted oil–butter with the remaining ingredients. Blend for 30 seconds, stop and repeat if needed.

3. Using a funnel, transfer to a spray bottle.

TO USE: Shake well, and then spray onto dry or damp hair.

STORAGE: Store in a cool, dry place for 2–5 months.

USE: As needed

TRY INSTEAD
If you don't have camellia oil on hand, use more argan in its place.

BEACH 'DO SPRAY

YIELD: ABOUT 2 OUNCES **TIME:** 30 MINUTES

GOOD FOR: ENHANCING NATURAL CURLS

With sea salt and aloe, this spray captures the essence of a day at the shore. It also contains hair-smoothing apple cider vinegar and vitamin E–rich palm oil. Because you melt the sea salt right into the green tea, you won't be left with salty sediment swimming in the bottom of the spray bottle.

FOR THE TEA:

1 cup water
1 bag green tea
½ tablespoon sea salt

FOR THE SPRAY:

⅛ teaspoon palm oil
¼ teaspoon apple cider vinegar
1 teaspoon aloe vera juice
¼ cup salt-tea mixture

1. On the stovetop in a small pot, heat the water until it's very hot, but not boiling. Add the teabag and simmer until the liquid is reduced by half. Remove the teabag, and add the salt and simmer until the salt melts or it is reduced in half again (¼ cup), cool.

2. On the stovetop in a small pot, melt the palm oil over low heat. Remove from the heat.

3. In a mini food processor or blender, combine ¼ cup salt-tea mixture, palm oil, and the remaining ingredients. Blend for 15–45 seconds.

4. Using a funnel, transfer to a spray bottle.

TO USE: Spritz on damp hair.

STORAGE: Store in the refrigerator for 2–3 weeks.

USE: As needed

REPAIR & MEND SPRAY

YIELD: ABOUT 2 OUNCES **TIME:** 30 MINUTES

GOOD FOR: DRY OR DAMAGED HAIR

This hair spray is great to use before you style, after you wash your hair, and as a treatment to keep breakage and frizz at bay.

FOR THE TEA:

1 cup distilled water

1 teaspoon dried lavender petals

1 teaspoon dried rosemary

1 teaspoon dried fenugreek

1 teaspoon mustard seed

FOR THE SPRAY:

¼ teaspoon jojoba oil

½ teaspoon glycerin

½ tablespoon aloe vera juice

⅛ teaspoon apple cider vinegar

¼ cup prepared tea

1. On the stovetop in a small pot, heat the water until it's very hot, but not boiling. Add the lavender, rosemary, fenugreek, and mustard seed, and simmer until the liquid is reduced by half. Strain the tea and cool.

2. In a bowl, combine the remaining ingredients and ¼ cup prepared tea. Mix well.

3. Using a funnel, transfer to a spray bottle.

TO USE: Shake well and spritz on dry or damp hair.

STORAGE: Store in the refrigerator for 1–2 weeks.

USE: As needed

SOFT-HOLD HAIR SPRAY

YIELD: ABOUT 3 OUNCES TIME: 30 MINUTES

GOOD FOR: ALL HAIR TYPES

When a friend's child spilled some apple juice on me, I noticed that, as it started to dry, it felt sticky on my hands and a lightbulb went off. I headed to the lab and worked on this formula; this recipe is the end results of lots of tweaks, tons of willing test subjects, and gallons and gallons of apple juice.

½ cup aloe vera juice
1½ tablespoons apple juice
¼ cup vodka
1 tablespoon glycerin
2 tablespoons Hair Tea (page 126)

1. In a bowl, combine all the ingredients and mix well.

2. Using a funnel, transfer to a spray bottle.

TO USE: Spritz on dry hair, whenever you would use a soft-hold hair spray.

STORAGE: Store in the refrigerator for 3–5 weeks.

USE: As needed

DE-FRIZZING SHINE SPRAY

YIELD: 2½ OUNCES **TIME:** 20 MINUTES

GOOD FOR: DRY OR FRIZZY HAIR

Most OTC hair sprays rely on synthetic polymers, like silicone or dimethicone, which actually block moisture from reaching the hair shaft, causing the hair to become dry and brittle. Even though it may look shiny and healthy on the outside, over time it causes frizz. This hair spray recipe de-frizzes, shines, and moisturizes hair cuticles.

½ tablespoon palm oil
2 tablespoons vodka
1 ¼ tablespoons glycerin
½ tablespoon camellia oil
½ tablespoon jojoba oil

1. On the stovetop in a small pot, melt the palm oil over low heat. Remove from the heat.

2. In a mini food processor, combine the remaining ingredients and the melted palm oil. Blend for 15–45 seconds.

3. Using a funnel, transfer to a spray bottle.

TO USE: Spritz on dry hair to get rid of frizz or add shine.

STORAGE: Store in cool dry place for 1–2 months.

USE: As needed

DID YOU KNOW?
Vodka works by using a weak acid (a low pH) to smooth the cuticle. Alcohol alone can be drying, but in combination with the other moisturizing ingredients, it helps smoothing.

BEER HAIR MASK

There's an old wives' tale suggesting that beer makes hair grow, enhances its thickness and shine, and is smoothing and softening. While there's no real evidence that beer aids in hair growth, the protein in beer does help strengthen hair cuticles, which sets the stage for hair growth.

1 egg white
1 egg yolk
½ cup beer
1 tablespoon apple cider vinegar
1 tablespoon Hair Tea (page 126)

1. In a bowl, whisk the egg white until stiff. Set aside.

2. In a mini food processor or blender, combine the remaining ingredients, and blend for 10 to 20 seconds.

3. In the bowl, fold the mixture into the egg white.

TO USE: Apply to your hair before you get into the shower. Cover your hair with a shower cap or plastic bag. Leave on for 5–30 minutes, then rinse and shampoo.

STORAGE: It's best to use this recipe very soon after you make it, but it will keep in the refrigerator for up to 1 week.

USE: As needed

TRY INSTEAD

If you're pressed for time, forego the full hair mask and just do a beer rinse. It is also an acid, which closes cuticles and works to smooth your hair's surface, which in turn makes it reflect light, giving it the appearance of shine. Any beer will do. Before shampooing, spray it on your hair or pour it right over your hair in the shower.

HONEY & AVOCADO HAIR MASK

YIELD: ABOUT 5 OUNCES **TIME:** 10 MINUTES

GOOD FOR: ALL HAIR TYPES

Honey helps moisturize hair, while the avocado, egg, and coconut milk contain essential fatty acids and proteins to keep your hair cuticles in good shape.

1 egg
⅛ avocado
¼ cup coconut milk
¼ cup Hair Tea (page 126)
1 tablespoon honey

1. In a mini food processor or blender, combine all the ingredients. Blend in 10- to 20- second intervals until the mixture is smooth.

2. Transfer to an airtight container.

TO USE: Apply to your hair with a wide-tooth comb before getting in the shower. Cover your hair with a shower cap or plastic bag. Leave the mask on for 5–30 minutes, then rinse and shampoo.

STORAGE: It's best to use this recipe very soon after you make it, but it will keep in the refrigerator for up to 1 week.

USE: As needed

LUSCIOUS LOCKS / HAIR MASKS

OLIVE, HEMP & COCONUT OIL HAIR

YIELD: 4½ OUNCES **TIME:** 20 MINUTES

GOOD FOR: ALL HAIR TYPES

Hemp oil is the star of this recipe. It's high in proteins that protect and help maintain healthy hair. The other ingredients are also star in their own right, providing their own array of hair-enhancing benefits.

¼ cup Hair Tea (page 126)
2 tablespoons aloe vera juice
1 teaspoon coconut oil
1 teaspoon olive oil
1 teaspoon hemp oil
1 teaspoon apple cider vinegar

In a mini food processor or blender, combine all the ingredients, and blend in 10- to 20-second intervals until the mixture is smooth.

TO USE: Apply to your hair with a wide-tooth comb before getting in the shower. Cover your hair with a shower cap or plastic bag. Leave on for 5–30 minutes, then rinse and shampoo. You may need to shampoo twice.

STORAGE: It's best to use this recipe very soon after you make it, but it will keep in the refrigerator for up to 1 week.

USE: As needed; recommended once per month for oily hair

DID YOU KNOW?

There is an open debate on whether or not the proteins we use in DIY products can penetrate the hair shaft as well as the hydrolyzed protein that is used in commercial shampoos and conditioner. Using a variety of different natural protein sources will help you determine which protein sources provide you with the most benefit—and you won't have to take your chances with the other ingredients found in OTC hair products.

5

LUSCIOUS LOCKS / HAIR MASKS

APPLE CIDER VINEGAR & LEMON HAIR MASK

YIELD: 10 OUNCES **TIME:** 20 MINUTES

GOOD FOR: OILY HAIR, CLEANING PRODUCT BUILDUP

The clarifying and acidic properties of apple cider vinegar, strawberries, and lemon make this mask ideal for a hair detox. Along with the clay, they'll help rid you of buildup on your scalp and strands. Remember to strain this one . . . you don't want any of those tiny strawberry seeds in your mane—they can be hard to locate!

½ cup apple cider vinegar
½ cup Hair Tea (page 126)
2 strawberries
1 tablespoon lemon juice
1 tablespoon kaolin clay

1. In a mini food processor or blender, combine all the ingredients, and blend in 10- to 20-second intervals until the mixture is smooth.

2. Pour mixture through a fine-mesh strainer, nut milk bag, or cheesecloth over a bowl or glass to strain out the strawberry seeds.

3. Transfer to an airtight container.

TO USE: Apply to your hair before getting in the shower. You can "dip" your hair into the mask or you can apply it with a toner bottle. Cover your hair with a shower cap or plastic bag. Leave on for 5–30 minutes, then rinse and shampoo.

STORAGE: Store in the refrigerator for up to 1 week.

USE: As needed

A CLOSER LOOK

Just like your pores need a deep cleaning every once in a while to stay healthy, so does your hair. Your natural oils mixed with dirt, pollution, chemicals, and polymers in hair-care products can leave a coating on the hair shaft and cause damage. How often you need to do a deep clean depends on your hair type and lifestyle (such as if you smoke or use a lot of products in your hair).

LUSCIOUS LOCKS / HAIR MASKS

5

BANANA, HONEY & MILK HAIR MASK

YIELD: ABOUT 2½ OUNCES **TIME:** 20 MINUTES

GOOD FOR: DRY HAIR, ITCHY SCALP

Rich in vitamins A, E, and C, as well as potassium, banana is a wonderful addition to hair masks. It is great for dry hair and itchy, flaky scalps, helping hydrate the hair along with the honey and coconut.

⅛ banana

⅛ teaspoon honey

⅛ teaspoon lecithin

1½ tablespoons yogurt

2 tablespoons rice milk

1 tablespoon coconut milk

OPTIONAL INGREDIENTS:

1 teaspoon egg (all hair types)

1 teaspoon apple cider vinegar (all hair types)

¼ teaspoon clay (oily hair)

¼ avocado (oily hair)

¼ to ½ teaspoon jojoba oil (dry hair)

⅛ teaspoon wheat germ oil (dry hair)

In a mini food processor, combine all the ingredients, and blend in 10- to 20-second intervals until mixture is smooth.

TO USE: Apply to your hair (with a wide-tooth comb if you choose) before getting in the shower. Cover your hair with a shower cap or plastic bag. Leave it on for 5 to 30 minutes, then rinse and shampoo.

STORAGE: It's best to use this recipe very soon after you make it, but it will keep in the refrigerator for up to 1 week.

USE: As needed

A CLOSER LOOK

When adding optional ingredients, keep an eye out for consistency. If your mask is too runny, you can apply it with a toner bottle, and if it's too thick, it might be difficult to spread. If necessary, add a little more of the dry or liquid ingredients to get a good consistency.

CAMELLIA ANTIFRIZZ HAIR MASK

YIELD: ¾ OUNCE **TIME:** 20 MINUTES

GOOD FOR: FRIZZ AND BREAKAGE

Camellia oil has moisturizing properties and also contains a high level of antioxidants. Combined with the other oils in this recipe, this amazing oil provides shine and helps correct the dryness that causes both frizz and breakage.

½ teaspoon palm oil

½ tablespoon camellia oil

½ tablespoon jojoba oil

¼ cup aloe vera juice

½ teaspoon glycerin

1. On the stovetop in a small pot, melt the palm oil over low heat. Remove from the heat.

2. In a mini food processor, combine the remaining ingredients and the melted palm oil. Blend for 15–45 seconds.

3. Transfer to an airtight container.

TO USE: Apply to your hair with a wide-tooth comb before getting in the shower. Cover your hair with a shower cap or plastic bag. Leave it on for 5–30 minutes, then rinse and shampoo. When using an oil mask, you may need to wash 2–3 times.

STORAGE: It's best to use this recipe very soon after you make it, but it will keep in the refrigerator for up to 1 week.

USE: As needed

DID YOU KNOW?

Camellia oil is derived from *Camellia sinensis*. This is the same plant from which the following teas are made: oolong, black, green, and white tea. Yes, these teas all come from the same plant!

COCONUT ANTIFRIZZ HAIR MASK

YIELD: 2 OUNCES **TIME:** 20 MINUTES

GOOD FOR: DRY HAIR, FRIZZ AND BREAKAGE

You may frequently see aloe contained in OTC hair products because it's great for the hair, helping to balance pH levels and smooth hair cuticles.

2 teaspoons coconut butter
2 teaspoons glycerin
¼ cup aloe vera gel

1. On the stovetop in a small pot, melt the coconut butter over low heat. Remove from the heat.

2. In a mini food processor, combine the remaining ingredients and melted coconut butter. Blend the mixture until smooth.

3. Transfer to an airtight container.

TO USE: Apply to your hair with a wide-tooth comb before getting in the shower. Cover your hair with a shower cap or plastic bag. Leave it on for 5–30 minutes, then rinse and shampoo.

STORAGE: It's best to use this recipe very soon after you make it, but it will keep in the refrigerator for up to 3 weeks.

USE: As needed

A CLOSER LOOK

Maintaining the pH of your skin, hair, and scalp is one of the most important things you can do. Your hair and scalp are similar to your skin in that they have a slightly acidic mantle that acts as a barrier, protecting against bacteria, viruses, and contamination. In small amounts, and not over a prolonged period, alkaline hair products can help aid in penetration by opening the cuticle. Acidic products harden the outside layer, flatten cuticles and shrink the diameter of the hair, making it less prone to tangles. You need products that encourage this opening and flattening process to maintain your luscious locks.

SLIPPERY ELM DETANGLER

YIELD: ABOUT 10 OUNCES **TIME:** 30 MINUTES

GOOD FOR: TANGLED HAIR

Slippery elm and Irish moss are natural sources of mucilage (a protein-rich, viscous substance), which provides the slip and glide needed to prevent tangles. Aloe vera helps balance pH levels and tighten the hair cuticles, but it can be omitted from the recipe if you don't have it on hand. You'll still get the detangling effects you're after.

FOR TEA:

2 cups Hair Tea (page 126)

¼ cup slippery elm root (do not use powdered if you can find cut and sift; the powders are much harder to strain)

3 tablespoons Irish moss (do not use powdered if you can find cut and sift)

FOR SPRAY:

¼ cup aloe vera juice

½ teaspoon glycerin

½ cup of tea

1. On the stovetop in a medium pot, combine the Hair Tea, slippery elm root, and Irish moss. Heat the water until it's hot, but not boiling. Turn the heat to low and simmer until the liquid is reduced by half. Strain the tea and cool.

2. In a small bowl, combine the aloe vera juice and glycerin with ½ cup of the tea mixture, and mix well.

3. Using a funnel, transfer to a spray bottle.

TO USE: Spray onto damp hair and gently comb through.

STORAGE: Store in the refrigerator for 1–2 weeks.

USE: As needed

DID YOU KNOW?

The detanglers you'll find on store shelves might provide the slip you want, but like many OTC conditioners, they coat the hair with synthetic polymers, oils, and acids. These synthetics might make your hair appear tight and smooth, but repeated use will damage the hair over time.

APPLE CIDER VINEGAR DETANGLER

YIELD: 2 OUNCES **TIME:** 15 MINUTES

GOOD FOR: TANGLED HAIR

Think of your hair cuticles as roof shingles; apple cider vinegar helps them lay flat so that the surface of your "roof" is smooth and attractive. This smoothening detangler also gives your hair wonderful shine.

⅛ cup apple cider vinegar
⅛ cup Hair Tea (page 126)
¼ teaspoon jojoba oil
¼ teaspoon glycerin

1. In a small bowl, combine all the ingredients and mix well.

2. Using a funnel, transfer to a spray bottle.

TO USE: Spray onto dry or damp hair and gently comb through.

STORAGE: Store in the refrigerator for 1–2 weeks.

USE: As needed

A CLOSER LOOK

Glycerin has a long and involved history—it is naturally produced during the saponification process (a chemical reaction between an acid and base to form a salt) when making soaps. During World War II, soap makers realized they could extract the natural glycosides and sell them to the weapons industry. What was left became the hard detergent bars we still use today. Real handmade soap is harder to find. This may lead you to think the clear glycerin bars you can purchase would be full all the goodness; however, pure glycerin is not clear, it is milky and viscous. To make it clear, it is put through an ethyl alcohol process, which is one of the reasons the glycerin soaps you buy in the store are not good for the skin. When pure glycerin is used in skin-care products in the proper amount, it can be a wonderful ingredient. It is a humectant, which helps skin retain moisture. However, if too much is used, it can pull the moisture from your skin.

BEESWAX & PALM OIL HAIR WAX

YIELD: 3½ OUNCES **TIME:** 40 MINUTES

GOOD FOR: ALL HAIR TYPES

Like gel or spray, hair wax can also be used to hold your style in place. Wax is not as drying as OTC gels and sprays. It will not damage the hair shaft. In fact, it moisturizes tresses and promotes healthy hair, while providing the control you want.

2 tablespoons beeswax

3 tablespoons palm oil

2 tablespoons jojoba oil

2 to 8 drops any essential oil (optional)

1. In a mini slow cooker or a double boiler that you've dedicated to beeswax products, melt the beeswax on low heat.

2. Once the beeswax is melted, add the palm oil and stir.

3. Add the remaining ingredients to the wax. Stir with a spoon that you've dedicated to beeswax products until well combined.

4. Transfer to an airtight container. The wax will be hot, so be mindful to pour it into heat-resistant containers. Silicone molds work well and make the wax easy to use.

TO USE: Warm a dime-size amount of the product in your hands. Apply to your hair and style as desired. If you make it in a mold, you can rub your hands with the wax and then apply from hands to hair.

STORAGE: Store in a cool, dry place for up to 1 year.

USE: As desired

A CLOSER LOOK

The addition of essential oils to a recipe can profoundly affect the way a product works. I recommend going light on these natural scents in the beginning to see if they change the efficacy of your product.

SHEA BUTTER HAIR WAX

YIELD: ABOUT 4 OUNCES **TIME:** 40 MINUTES

GOOD FOR: ALL HAIR TYPES, ESPECIALLY DRY HAIR

This wax is a little richer and higher in essential fatty acids than the previous one. If you have very dry, brittle hair, you may prefer this hair wax. On the other hand, if you tend to have oily hair, you may find the other wax more to your liking.

3½ tablespoons beeswax
2 tablespoons coconut butter
1 tablespoon glycerin
2 tablespoons shea butter

1. In a mini slow cooker or a double boiler that you've dedicated to beeswax products, melt the beeswax on low heat.

2. Add the coconut butter and glycerin to the wax. Stir with a spoon that you've dedicated to beeswax products until well combined.

3. Add the shea butter, stir, and remove from the heat.

4. Transfer to an airtight container or silicone molds and put it in the freezer till completely cooled.

TO USE: Warm a dime-size amount of the product in your hands. Apply to hair and style as desired. If you make it in a mold, you can rub your hands with the wax and then apply from hands to hair.

STORAGE: Store in a cool, dry place for up to 1 year.

USE: As desired

DID YOU KNOW?
There's an added bonus to hair wax! It will also moisturize your hands and cuticles. Try massaging some into your cuticles as needed.

5

LUSCIOUS LOCKS / HAIR WAXES

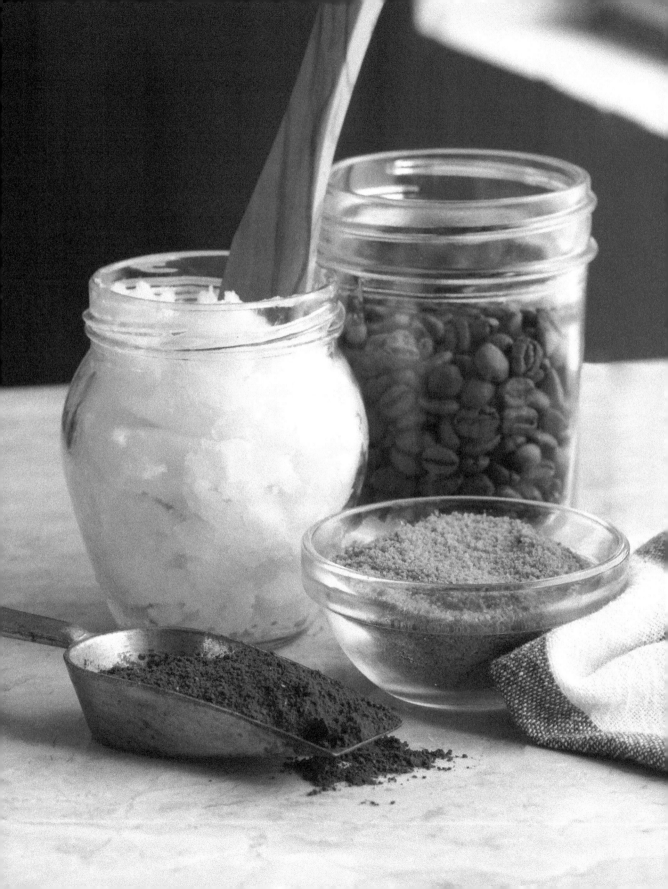

6
POTPOURRI

Throughout the book I've included some of my favorite recipes to make with friends—and kids! In this chapter you'll find head-to-toe recipes to keep your teeth, nails, and feet healthy. These DIY products are fun to make. Some of them make the perfect at-home spa products for having an impromptu spa day: Mix up the products, apply them, and then settle in for a great chat while the active ingredients hydrate and smooth your skin.

ARROWROOT & BAKING
SODA TOOTHPASTE

YIELD: ABOUT 2 OUNCES **TIME:** 15 MINUTES

GOOD FOR: ORAL HYGIENE

Baking soda has long been incorporated into DIY toothpaste mixtures for its deep-cleaning properties. Including arrowroot in this toothpaste helps cut the abrasiveness of the baking soda. It's always nice when toothpaste leaves your mouth with a pleasant, fresh taste, so feel free to add a little natural flavoring, like peppermint or spearmint.

⅛ cup arrowroot

⅛ cup baking soda* (or orris root, for sensitive teeth)

1½ teaspoons glycerin

2 to 10 drops flavoring**

1 drop hydrogen peroxide* (optional, for whitening)

* *Check with your dentist to make sure baking soda and hydrogen peroxide are right for you.*

** *Not all essential oils are good for internal use— check the packaging on the brands you buy. To flavor toothpaste you can use anything you'd use to cook or bake with, like vanilla or mint.*

1. In a small bowl, combine arrowroot and baking soda (or orris root) and mix well.

2. Add the remaining ingredients, and mix again until well combined.

3. Transfer to an airtight container.

TO USE: Sprinkle some of the powder on your toothbrush. Keep in mind that it won't foam as much as commercial products.

STORAGE: Store for 2–4 months in the refrigerator, or 1–2 weeks at room temperature.

USE: Twice daily

A CLOSER LOOK

In recent years, there has been some controversy over whether baking soda is suitable for daily use on our enamel due to its abrasiveness. Before you begin using either baking soda or orris root regularly, ask your dentist for advice. Orris root can be used instead, which is less abrasive but still debatable.

ARROWROOT & COCONUT BUTTER TOOTHPASTE

YIELD: ABOUT 4 OUNCES **TIME:** 25 MINUTES

GOOD FOR: ORAL HYGIENE

I interviewed several dentists to get their thoughts on homemade tooth-pastes, and we discussed the best ingredients to use for maximum cleansing and maintenance. After much research and many attempts at a formula, this recipe was born.

6 tablespoons coconut butter
½ cup arrowroot
3 teaspoons glycerin
1 drop peppermint oil

1. On the stovetop in a small pot, melt the coconut butter over low heat. Remove from the heat.

2. Add the glycerin, and mix well.

3. Add the arrowroot and mix well.

4. Add the peppermint oil, and mix well.

5. Transfer to an airtight container.

TO USE: Use as you would any other toothpaste. Keep in mind that it won't foam as much as commercial products.

STORAGE: Store for 2–4 months in the refrigerator or 1–2 weeks at room temperature.

USE: Twice daily

SUNFLOWER & SESAME OIL PULL

YIELD: 2 OUNCES **TIME:** 5 MINUTES

GOOD FOR: ORAL HYGIENE

Sunflower and sesame seed oils are traditionally touted as the best oil-pulling solution. Though coconut is often a go-to for oil pulls, some people don't like the taste of coconut. If you're one of them, this is the recipe for you.

2 tablespoons sesame oil

2 tablespoons sunflower oil

1 drop essential oil of clove, cinnamon, peppermint, myrrh, lemon, or rosemary (do not use one drop of each in the same mixture!)*

* *Not all essential oils are good for internal use— check the packaging on the brands you buy.*

1. In a small bowl, combine the sesame and sunflower oils. Mix well.

2. Add the essential oil, and mix again.

3. Transfer to an airtight container.

TO USE: After brushing, swish 1 tablespoon of oil mixture in your mouth for 5–20 minutes. To save time, oil pull while you shower.

STORAGE: Store in the refrigerator for 3–5 months.

USE: 3 times per week

DID YOU KNOW?

Oil pulling is an oral-cleansing routine in Ayurvedic medicine, a holistic health-care system with roots in ancient India. Proponents of oil pulling maintain that the oil attracts bacteria and other toxins in the mouth, which are then expelled when the oil is spit out. It is recommended that oil pulling be practiced after brushing and on an empty stomach. It's also a good idea to rinse your mouth out with water afterward. You don't have to start with the full 20 minutes. Some people start by swishing for 5 minutes and work their way up to the full 20 minutes. The dentists I consulted had favorable opinions of this routine, but oil pulling should not be substituted for regular oral health care and dental visits.

COCONUT BUTTER OIL PULL

YIELD: 2 OUNCES TIME: 10 MINUTES

GOOD FOR: ORAL HYGIENE

Because of its known antibacterial properties, coconut butter is a natural pick for oil pulling. Fifty percent of the fat in coconut butter is made of lauric acid, which is known for its antimicrobial properties. Look for virgin coconut butter for the best results.

¼ cup coconut butter

2 drops of essential oil of clove, cinnamon, peppermint, myrrh, lemon, or rosemary (optional; do not use one drop of each in the same mixture!)∗

∗ Not all essential oils are good for internal use—check the packaging on the brands you buy.

1. On the stovetop in a small pot, melt the coconut butter over low heat. Remove from the heat.

2. Add the essential oil, if using, to the melted butter. Stir to mix.

3. Pour into single-use molds that can hold 1 tablespoon of fluid. Plastic chocolate molds work well. There are all kinds of little cavity molds such as flowers, thin circles, and shapes. You can find them where you would buy chocolate-making supplies, at some craft stores or baking stores.

TO USE: After brushing, swish 1 tablet (whatever shape mold you used) in your mouth for 5–20 minutes. The coconut butter will liquefy with the heat of your mouth, but the molded shapes make the single-serve portions easy to use. To save time, oil pull while you shower.

STORAGE: Store in the refrigerator for up to 3–5 months.

USE: 3 times per week

A CLOSER LOOK

The essential oils recommended in this recipe all have oral hygiene benefits—from promoting gum health to freshening your breath. Because essential oils have their own efficacies and can be caustic when too much is used, add no more than 2 drops per ¼ cup of coconut butter.

BAKING SODA MOUTHWASH

YIELD: ABOUT 16 OUNCES **TIME:** 15 MINUTES

GOOD FOR: ORAL HYGIENE

This simple mouthwash offers the cleansing benefits of baking soda in a gentler form than brushing and doesn't contain the alcohol that's found in most OTC mouthwashes. Give this mouthwash a good swish to get it into all the nooks and crannies in your teeth and gums.

2 cups peppermint hydrosol or distilled water

1 tablespoon baking soda

2 drops essential oil of cinnamon, tea tree, lemon, or peppermint (optional)∗

∗ *Not all essential oils are good for internal use—check the packaging on the brands you buy.*

1. In a medium bowl, combine all the ingredients and mix well.

2. Using a funnel, transfer to an airtight container.

TO USE: After brushing your teeth, swish 1 tablespoon around your mouth.

STORAGE: Store in the refrigerator for up to 4 weeks.

USE: As needed

DID YOU KNOW?

There's some debate over whether alcohol is actually necessary in mouthwash to maintain good oral health. While it does reduce the bacteria and buildup between teeth, it doesn't necessarily promote overall health. In your DIY products, there's no need to add it. Your mouth will get clean without it.

APPLE CIDER VINEGAR MOUTHWASH

YIELD: 4 OUNCES **TIME:** 10 MINUTES

GOOD FOR: ORAL HYGIENE

Apple cider vinegar helps break down plaque and kill bacteria. It's important to note that apple cider vinegar is an acid, and overuse will break down the enamel on your teeth, which is why I recommend diluting it with lavender hydrosol and using it only once a month for deep cleaning.

¼ cup apple cider vinegar
¼ cup lavender hydrosol

1. In a small bowl, combine the ingredients and mix well.

2. Using a funnel, transfer to an airtight container.

TO USE: After brushing, swish 1 tablespoon in your mouth, then rinse well with water.

STORAGE: Store in the refrigerator for up to 4 weeks.

USE: As needed

DID YOU KNOW?

In addition to its antibacterial and infection-fighting properties, lavender also stimulates circulation and aids in digestion. This makes it a great ingredient in oral-care recipes. Its calming, relaxing scent is an added bonus.

BUTTER & OIL CUTICLE TREATMENT

YIELD: ABOUT 1¼ OUNCES **TIME:** 20 MINUTES

GOOD FOR: ALL SKIN TYPES

We use our hands all day, every day, and they never complain—even though they tend to age faster than other parts of our body and need special care. Dryness, hangnails, brittle nails, inflamed cuticles, and itchy, flaky skin are among the common complaints for both hands and nails. While many women leave nail care only for when they have time for the salon, a little oil applied at home can keep cuticles and nails healthy.

2 teaspoons coconut butter
3 teaspoons shea butter
1 teaspoon apricot oil
1 teaspoon avocado oil
⅛ teaspoon tamanu oil
⅛ teaspoon hemp oil

1. On the stovetop in a small pot, melt the coconut butter over low heat. Remove from the heat.

2. Add the shea butter to the coconut butter, and mix well. (The warmth from the coconut butter should be enough to melt it.)

3. Add the remaining ingredients to the butter mixture, and mix again.

4. Transfer to an airtight container and put in the freezer immediately till completely cooled.

TO USE: Dab a little bit of the oil onto the cuticles and massage in.

STORAGE: Store in a cool, dry place for 3–5 months.

USE: As needed

DID YOU KNOW?

Oil penetrates faster and deeper than lotions and creams. I teach my clients a technique for dry skin (on both body and face) that I call "seal the deal." First apply a face or body oil and then a lotion or cream to lock in the moisture and seal the deal. This simple layering technique has a huge impact and vastly improves dry skin.

GOAT MILK & AVOCADO HAND SOAK

YIELD: ABOUT 1 USE **TIME:** 15 MINUTES

GOOD FOR: DRY SKIN, SOFTENING AND YELLOWING NAILS

A nourishing hand soak is a great way to soften your skin while both cleansing and preparing your hands for absorbing moisture afterward. This blend is particularly excellent for dealing with dry hands. The lemon juice will help with yellowing nails, too. Be sure the baking soda, milk, and oil mixture is thoroughly blended before adding the lemon juice, to avoid curdling.

1 tablespoon baking soda
1 teaspoon goat milk
⅛ teaspoon avocado oil
1 drop lemon essential oil
1 drop tea tree or lavender essential oil
½ tablespoon lemon juice

1. In a small bowl, combine the baking soda, goat milk, and oils. Mix well.

2. Add the lemon juice, and mix again.

3. Use immediately.

TO USE: In a bowl that's large enough to fully submerge your hands, combine 2–4 cups of warm water (the amount will depend on the size and shape of your bowl) and the hand soak mixture. Stir to mix. Soak your hands for 5–15 minutes. Pat dry.

STORAGE: Use immediately.

USE: As desired

A CLOSER LOOK

You don't have to wait for your next trip to the salon for a professional manicure. You can give yourself one! Start by trimming and filing your nails, follow up with a scrub and a soak, and then massage lotion and cuticle oil, gently pushing back your cuticles. Wash your nails thoroughly to remove oil and lotion in preparation for polishing.

COCONUT HAND SCRUB & MASK

YIELD: ABOUT 4 OUNCES TIME: 20 MINUTES

GOOD FOR: ALL SKIN TYPES

A hand scrub can help exfoliate skin while leaving hands smooth and moisturized. This coconut blend is perfect for using up the last little bits of coconut in your pantry... or anytime you want to have a spa experience at home. If you have some extra time, follow the instructions for making a nourishing hand mask.

¼ cup coconut flour
¼ cup coconut sugar
½ tablespoon coconut butter
1 teaspoon cocoa butter
1½ tablespoons coconut milk*

* *To make this scrub into a hand mask you will need to add 6 more tablespoons of the coconut milk*

1. In a small bowl, combine the coconut flour and sugar, and mix well. Set aside.

2. On the stovetop in a small pot, melt the coconut butter and cocoa butter over low heat. Remove from the heat.

3. Add the melted butters to the dry mixture, and mix well.

4. Add the coconut milk, and mix again until thoroughly incorporated.

5. Transfer to an airtight container.

TO USE AS A HAND SCRUB: Wash and dry your hands. Work a dime-size amount of the scrub over your hands for 15 to 20 seconds, then rinse off and pat dry. You want the ingredients to stay on your skin, so there's no need to wash your hands after using the scrub; a simple rinse will do.

TO USE AS A MASK: For the hand mask: You'll need one plastic bag for each hand. (I find that produce bags work best.) Place half the mixture in each bag, slip your hand in, and work the scrub around your fingers and hand. Leave the bag on for 5–15 minutes. If you're alone, do one hand at a time, or get a friend to help you so that you can do both hands at once.

STORAGE: Store in the refrigerator for 1–2 weeks.

USE: As desired

CLAY & POLENTA FOOT SCRUB & MASK

YIELD: 6½ OUNCES (2 USES FOR BOTH FEET) **TIME:** 10 MINUTES

GOOD FOR: DRY SKIN; ROUGH HEELS; OR ACHY, TIRED FEET.

Foot masks make a fun activity to do during girls' nights in or a DIY spa party, with your partner or family members. When you have a lot of people, you can make a big batch of this clay-coconut scrub, but be sure to have two plastic bags for everyone. It might take a while to get used to having bags on your feet, but the softening, healing, soothing, and relaxing effects of this mask are worth it.

¼ cup kaolin clay
¼ cup bentonite clay
¼ cup arrowroot
1 tablespoon organic polenta
About 3 tablespoons coconut milk (enough to make a paste)

GIFT IT

Invite a few friends over for a spa party and prepare the foot masks and hand masks before everyone arrives. Although it's fun to make DIY products together, preparing the mixtures ahead of time allows you and your friends to get right down to your body-care basics.

1. In a medium bowl, combine the clays, arrowroot, and polenta, and mix well.

2. Add 1 tablespoon at a time of coconut milk to make a paste. (It should be about the consistency of a smoothie.)

3. Transfer to an airtight container.

TO USE AS A FOOT SCRUB: Wash feet. Depending on the size of your feet, you'll need between ½ tablespoon and 1 tablespoon of the scrub per foot. Massage the scrub into your feet (you can do it over the bathtub, or a hand towel to prevent a mess). Rinse off under running water. You want the ingredients to stay on your skin, so there's no need to wash your feet after using the scrub; a simple rinse will do.

TO USE AS A FOOT MASK: For the mask, you'll need one plastic bag for each foot. (I find that produce bags work best.) Place half the mixture in each bag, slip it on your foot, and work the scrub around your toes and foot. Leave the bags on for 5–15 minutes.

STORAGE: Store in the refrigerator for 1–2 weeks.

USE: As desired

TEA TREE FOOT SOAK

YIELD: 11 OUNCES **TIME:** 15 MINUTES

GOOD FOR: SOFTENING, SOOTHING ACHY TIRED FEET, ALLEVIATING ROUGH HEELS

This blend of salts, hydrosols, and vinegar tackles so many tootsie issues at once. From dealing with everything from odor to roughness, this formula will become a fast favorite—especially during sandal season and the cold season when hibernating feet can become excessively dry.

¼ cup tea tree hydrosol

¼ cup lavender hydrosol

¼ cup rosemary hydrosol

¼ cup apple cider vinegar

2 tablespoons sea salt

2 tablespoons Epsom salt

2 tablespoons baking soda

5 drops of essential oil of lavender, cassia, lemon, sweet orange, rosemary, clove, tea tree, or mint (optional; do not use 5 drops of each)

1. Warm the hydrosols.

2. Have some warm water at the ready if you need it.

3. In a large bowl that's large enough to fully submerge your feet, combine all the dry ingredients, and mix well.

TO USE: Have your warm water at the ready and put your feet in the bowl. Add enough of the warm water to cover your feet and swish to mix. Make sure not to pour the warm water directly on your feet. Soak your feet for 5–15 minutes. Pat dry.

STORAGE: Use immediately.

USE: As desired

TRY INSTEAD

If you are struggling with foot fungus, this foot soak can be personalized for your needs by adding ingredients with antifungal properties. Prepare the soak as directed, leaving out the optional essential oils and use instead: 2 drops of oregano essential oil, 2 drops of olive leaf extract, and 4 drops tamanu oil. Your feet and nails will thank you!

POTPOURRI / FOOT CARE

6

COCONUT, COCOA & TAMANU FOOT BUTTER

YIELD: ABOUT 4 OUNCES TIME: 30 MINUTES

GOOD FOR: ROUGH HEELS, DRY SKIN

Our hands and feet have fewer sebaceous glands than other areas of our skin, which is why we often struggle with dryness when it comes to these all-important parts of our bodies. This rich butter will keep your feet hydrated and soft, letting them know how much you appreciate all they do for you!

⅛ cup coconut butter
¼ cup cocoa butter
⅛ cup shea butter
½ tablespoon tamanu oil
2 drops lavender essential oil
1 drop peppermint essential oil

1. On the stovetop in a small pot, melt the coconut butter and the cocoa butter over low heat. Remove from the heat.

2. Add the shea butter to the melted butters. (The warmth from the melted butters should be enough to melt the shea butter.) Mix well.

3. Add the remaining oils to the butter mixture, and mix again.

4. Transfer to an airtight container and put in the freezer immediately till it is cooled.

TO USE: Massage a dime-size amount of butter onto each foot.

STORAGE: Store in an airtight container for 3–5 months.

USE: As desired

DRY SKIN SOLUTIONS

Does your skin feel excessively dry even though you've tried virtually everything to keep the moisture in? If you find yourself struggling with this issue, give the following tips a try:

1. Take warm (not hot!) baths and showers using butter-rich scrubs and moisturizers. Pat dry; avoid rough rubbing.

2. Avoid soaking in chemical-laden bubble baths and other bath products; avoid using synthetically fragrant and detergent-based soaps. Chemicals are not allies when combating some skin issues. Harsh detergents strip the skin when washing, and the alcohols and chemicals in creams and lotions further dry out the skin. Switch to hand-made, chemical-free soaps and moisturizers to really care for your skin.

3. Your body loses most of the moisture within 5 minutes of getting out of the bath or shower. To combat this, apply moisturizer right after you're done bathing or use a scrub in the shower to reduce the loss.

4. Drink your "eight by eight" (that's 8 ounces of water 8 times a day) while avoiding alcohol and caffeine-containing beverages, which act as diuretics.

5. If you are taking medication regularly, find out how it might affect your skin. If you know what you're up against, you can combat the side effects.

6. Limit your sun exposure—and don't forget your feet when you apply sunblock.

7. If you spend a lot of time in air-conditioned or heated rooms, get a humidifier, which adds much-needed moisture back into the air.

8. For dry feet, wear shoes that will help your feet breathe—like leather sneakers and boots, or canvas shoes—and wear cotton socks.

9. For winter-weary hands, wear gloves to protect your hands from the cold, and moisturize them before and after going outside.

10. Scrub your feet to prevent buildup of dead skin cells and moisturize twice per day, no matter the season.

ROSEMARY, CEDAR & LAVENDER BAR DEODORANT

YIELD: ABOUT 10 OUNCES **TIME:** 30 MINUTES

This recipe is teen tested and mother approved! I actually came up with this formula when I discovered that my daughter was hiding her conventional deodorant from me. She couldn't find a natural deodorant that worked well enough for her, and since she was a teen in high school, she wasn't willing to smell bad to please her mom's chemical-free obsession. I knew I could make a deodorant that would be both acceptable and healthy for her, so I got right to the lab. We had a ton of trial runs before my smelly, sporty teenager gave this bar her blessing.

⅛ teaspoon fine grain salt

3 teaspoons baking soda

3 teaspoons arrowroot

3 ounces beeswax

4½ ounces safflower oil

3 drops rosemary essential oil

1 drop cedar essential oil

2 drops lavender essential oil

1. In a mini food processor, combine the salt and baking soda, and pulse until the mixture is powder smooth.

2. In a small bowl, combine the arrowroot and the salt–baking soda mixture, and mix well. Set aside.

3. In a mini slow cooker or double boiler that you've dedicated to beeswax products, melt the beeswax.

4. Add the oils to the melted beeswax in the slow cooker, and mix with a spoon that you've dedicated to beeswax products.

5. Add the beeswax–oil mixture to the bowl with the dry mixture, and mix again. The coolness of the powder mixture may start to solidify the waxes, but keep mixing until it's completely blended.

6. Pour into silicone or plastic molds and chill in the refrigerator or freezer until solid.

TO USE: Smooth on underarms the way you would OTC stick deodorants.

STORAGE: Store in a tin for 3–5 months.

USE: Daily

ROSEMARY, LEMON, CEDAR & SAGE SPRAY DEODORANT

YIELD: ABOUT 8 OUNCES **TIME:** 20 MINUTES

There are several factors when it comes to body odor. Most people are surprised to find out it is not the sweat itself that smells, but the bacteria that lives on our skin. So to reduce the odor, you have to neutralize the bacteria. The ingredients in this deodorant "eat" odor and "kill" bacteria.

¼ cup apple cider vinegar
¼ cup cedar hydrosol
¼ cup rosemary hydrosol
¼ cup witch hazel hydrosol
¼ teaspoon Dead Sea salts
¼ teaspoon Epsom salts
¼ teaspoon sea salt
2 drops lemon essential oil
1 drop cedar essential oil
1 drop sage essential oil

1. In a medium bowl, combine all the ingredients and mix well. Wait until the salts dissolve before bottling. If they are not dissolving, you can warm the mixture up.

2. Using a funnel, transfer to a spray bottle.

TO USE: Spray a few squirts under each arm.

STORAGE: Store in an airtight container in the refrigerator for 2–4 months.

USE: Daily

A CLOSER LOOK

Hydrosols (floral waters) are one of my many obsessions. They have all the properties and benefits of essential oils, including the scent, but they are not caustic like the oils, and are also more affordable. Two of my favorites are rose water and neroli water—they maintain the aromatherapeutic effects of oils, but with added benefits. Rose soothes crankiness, while neroli is great for treating stress and anxiety. On skin, rose water does wonders for anti-aging, and neroli is best used for reducing redness. Do note there are many things on the market labeled "plant water," "floral water," and "rose water." Most are nothing more than distilled (or even tap water) with a few drops of fragrance or essential oil. Look for products labeled plant distillates or hydrosols.

FLORAL ESSENTIAL OIL PERFUME

YIELD: ABOUT ⅛ TEASPOON WITHOUT CARRIER OIL **TIME:** 20 MINUTES

This is a subtle floral blend that combines the sweetness of orange, the earthiness of lavender, and the forwardness of bright jasmine. Even if floral scents aren't your favorite, you'll probably enjoy this balanced blend.

8 drops palmarosa essential oil
4 drops lavender essential oil
4 drops sweet orange essential oil
4 drops jasmine absolute
Jojoba or sunflower oil (as desired)

1. Drip the oils directly into a perfume roller bottle, atomizer, or other small glass bottle with a cap.

2. Add the jojoba oil or sunflower oil to the bottle in small increments until you reach the scent's desired strength.

3. Reinsert the roller (if using) and cap tightly. Shake the bottle to mix.

TO USE: Apply to pulse points, or wherever you'd like.

STORAGE: Store in an airtight container for 4–8 months. If storing in plastic, make sure it's PET plastic or a harder plastic that is safe for storing essential oils—high concentrations of essential oils can dissolve plastic over a long period of time.

USE: As desired

A CLOSER LOOK

After all the comments I have peppered throughout this book that too much essential oil can be caustic, you may wonder why I'm including these essential oil–blended perfumes. To be clear, essential oils are better than synthetic fragrances, and many of my clients love using essential oils for the amazing scents. I always suggest using perfumes in moderation. Just a dab of the DIY perfumes will do the trick!

SPICY ESSENTIAL OIL PERFUME

YIELD: ABOUT ⅛ TEASPOON WITHOUT CARRIER OIL TIME: 20 MINUTES

This spicy scent is reminiscent of the autumn. It mixes the creamy, comforting sweetness of vanilla with warm spicy notes of cinnamon and cardamom. A kiss of tangerine balances it all out.

6 drops cardamom essential oil
6 drops tangerine essential oil
6 drops vanilla absolute
2 drops cinnamon bark essential oil
Jojoba or sunflower oil (as desired)

1. Drip the oils directly into a perfume roller bottle, atomizer, or other small glass bottle with a cap.

2. Add the jojoba oil or sunflower oil to the bottle in small increments until you reach the scent's desired strength.

3. Reinsert the roller (if using) and cap tightly. Shake the bottle to mix.

TO USE: Apply to pulse points, or wherever you'd like.

STORAGE: Store in the roller or other container for 4–8 months.

USE: As desired

TRY INSTEAD
The yield of the essential oil blend is intentionally small in these recipes. If you love a particular scent, you can increase it by doubling, tripling, or even quadrupling the number of drops. Just make sure you use a large enough bottle to add a sufficient amount of carrier oil.

SWEET & SASSY ESSENTIAL OIL PERFUME

YIELD: ABOUT ⅜ TEASPOON WITHOUT CARRIER OIL TIME: 20 MINUTES

The name of this fan-favorite recipe says it all. This recipe yields more than the other perfume recipes to make room for just a single drop of playful patchouli—a "hippy-smelling" scent that would otherwise overpower the perfume. The patchouli combined with the sassy tang of sweet citrus and warm vanilla makes this a perfect everyday uplifting blend.

24 drops grapefruit essential oil
16 drops vanilla absolute
8 drops orange essential oil
8 drops lemon essential oil
1 drop patchouli essential oil
Jojoba or sunflower oil (as desired)

1. Drip the oils directly into a perfume roller bottle, atomizer, or other small glass bottle with a cap.

2. Add the jojoba oil or sunflower oil to the bottle in small increments until you reach the scent's desired strength.

3. Reinsert the roller (if using) and cap tightly. Shake the bottle to mix.

TO USE: Apply to pulse points, or wherever you'd like.

STORAGE: Store in an airtight container for 4–8 months.

USE: As desired

A CLOSER LOOK

If you don't want to use essential oils on your skin, you can apply a few drops to small piece of cloth, which you can keep in your pocket or purse, and take out when the mood strikes you.

6

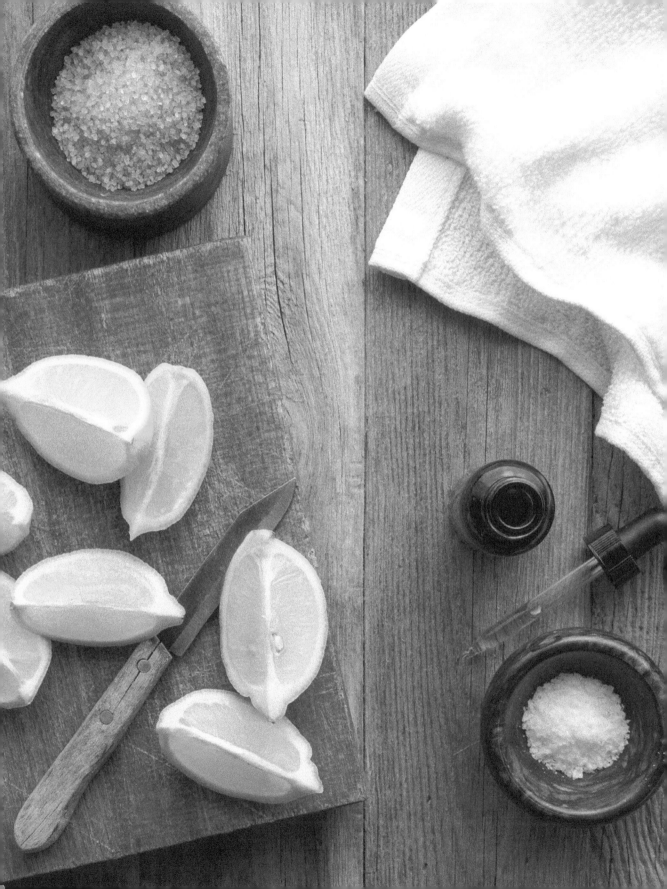

SAMPLE WEEKLY REGIMENS

Here you'll find a few sample weekly regimens based on your skin type. (See page 14 for descriptions of skin types.) Try these regimens at the start of your DIY skin-care journey. As you practice more and begin to see results, feel free to change up your routine. Skin actually responds well when you alter your routine at least once a year.

DRY SKIN

MORNING AND EVENING: Wash with Coconut Cleanser (page 55), follow up with Cucumber Toner (page 64), and finish with Macadamia, Kukui Nut & Avocado Moisturizer (page 75). Once daily, while in the shower, apply Goat Milk, Avocado & Honey Mask (page 82).

TWICE A WEEK: Switch out your mask for Pumpkin, Coconut & Brown Sugar Mask (page 83).

If skin is persistently dry, add Hydrating Serum (page 96) after toning, but before moisturizing.

NORMAL SKIN

MORNING AND EVENING: Wash with Strawberry, Honey & Oat Cleanser (page 50), follow up with Cucumber, Lemon & Tea Toner (page 71) or, to help smooth out wrinkles, Rose Hip & Citrus Toner (page 70). Complete your routine with Argan, Carrot & Sesame Moisturizer (page 73).

ONCE A WEEK, WHILE IN THE SHOWER: Avocado, Yogurt & Brewer's Yeast Mask (page 76).

COMBINATION SKIN

MORNING AND EVENING: Wash with Honey & Chia Seed Cleanser (page 57) and follow up with Tea & Vinegar Detox Toner (page 69). Finish with Argan, Carrot & Sesame Moisturizer (page 73).

ONCE A WEEK: Dead Sea Mud, Kombucha & Brewer's Yeast Mask (page 81).

OILY SKIN

MORNING AND EVENING: Wash with Activated Charcoal Cleanser (page 52) and follow up with Apple Juice, Sparkling Wine & Beer Toner (page 68) and St. John's Wort, Hemp & Avocado Moisturizer (page 74).

ONCE OR TWICE A WEEK: While in the shower, apply Turmeric, Yogurt & Honey Mask (page 79).

MATURE SKIN

MORNING AND EVENING: Wash with Hemp Cleanser (page 60) and follow up with Rose Hip & Citrus Toner (page 70). Finish with St. John's Wort, Hemp & Avocado Moisturizer (page 74).

ONCE OR TWICE A WEEK: While in the shower, apply Paprika, Honey & Buttermilk Mask (page 78).

Here are a few additional guidelines:

- Be sure to detox your skin at least once a year.
- If you have very oily or dry skin and are not getting the results you want, clean your pores. Do a deep-pore cleaning and use detox products for a month. Also pay close attention to other products you use that come in contact with your face, like shampoo and conditioner. Some OTC brands include ingredients that can clog and congest pores.
- If you have blemishes, do not exfoliate unless the recipe indicates it is for blemished skin.
- Start using the anti-aging products at the first signs of wrinkles.
- Skin can change types and needs over the course of your life, so keep up with your skin needs, not your skin image.

MORE INFORMATION ON SEEKING SAFE INGREDIENTS

It's very important to dig into the labels of any lotions or potions you are thinking of buying or already have on hand. The fronts of beauty bottles are often filled with claims about the product within, but the back is where you can find out if a product is in line with your criteria of what you deem safe and acceptable.

To find out what an ingredient is and if it's harmful, a good resource is the Material Data Safety Sheet (MSDS), which can be found online. This document provides health and safety information about substances, products, and chemicals. This is the same information and guidelines used by chemists when working with or handling these ingredients and it is provided to manufacturers and the consumer as well. Below is a list of ingredients I try to avoid (adapted and updated from my book *Look Great, Live Green*).

INGREDIENTS TO AVOID:
- Diethanolamine (DEA)
- Formaldehyde
- Nanoparticles
- Parabens
- Petroleum
- Phthalates
- Propylene glycol
- PVP/VA copolymer
- Synthetic fragrances
- Triethanolamine (TEA)

INGREDIENTS TO LOOK FOR:
- Arrowroot, in place of talc powder
- Colorants from minerals, to replace synthetic dyes
- Edible ingredients from your kitchen (honey, oatmeal, avocado, etc.)
- Essential oils instead of fragrance
- Extracts that list what they are extracted in, such "green tea extracted in organic grape alcohol"
- Fragrance-free products
- Nonfoaming facial cleansers and non-detergent body cleansers
- Powdered products, hard bar lotions that are made without water (which require less preservation and, therefore, fewer chemicals)
- Pure butters, such as shea and coconut
- Pure oils, like avocado, jojoba, and olive

MEASUREMENT CONVERSIONS

VOLUME EQUIVALENTS (LIQUID)

US STANDARD	US STANDARD (OUNCES)	METRIC (APPROXIMATE)
2 tablespoons	1 fl. oz.	30 mL
¼ cup	2 fl. oz.	60 mL
½ cup	4 fl. oz.	120 mL
1 cup	8 fl. oz.	240 mL
1½ cups	12 fl. oz.	355 mL
2 cups or 1 pint	16 fl. oz.	475 mL
4 cups or 1 quart	32 fl. oz.	1 L
1 gallon	128 fl. oz.	4 L

VOLUME EQUIVALENTS (DRY)

US STANDARD	METRIC (APPROXIMATE)
⅛ teaspoon	0.5 mL
¼ teaspoon	1 mL
½ teaspoon	2 mL
¾ teaspoon	4 mL
1 teaspoon	5 mL
1 tablespoon	15 mL
¼ cup	59 mL
⅓ cup	79 mL
½ cup	118 mL
⅔ cup	156 mL
¾ cup	177 mL
1 cup	235 mL
2 cups or 1 pint	475 mL
3 cups	700 mL
4 cups or 1 quart	1 L

OVEN TEMPERATURES

FAHRENHEIT (F)	CELSIUS (C) (APPROXIMATE)
250°F	120°C
300°F	150°C
325°F	165°C
350°F	180°C
375°F	190°C
400°F	200°C
425°F	220°C
450°F	230°C

WEIGHT EQUIVALENTS

US STANDARD	METRIC (APPROXIMATE)
½ ounce	15 g
1 ounce	30 g
2 ounces	60 g
4 ounces	115 g
8 ounces	225 g
12 ounces	340 g
16 ounces or 1 pound	455 g

RECIPE INDEX

INDEX

cedar hydrosol, 168
cell phones, 19
chamomile flowers, 93, 106
chamomile tea, 35, 69, 71
charcoals, 43
cheesecloth, 29
chemicals in skin-care products, 17–19, 24
chemistry, 9
chia seeds, 35, 57
cinnamon, 35, 99, 113
cinnamon bark essential oil, 41, 170
cinnamon essential oil, 41, 156–158
citric acid, 25, 35–36, 121–123
citrus essential oils, 114
citrus juice, 84, 114
citrus rind, 84, 94, 114
clays, 43, 83, 85, 145
cleansers, 21
    coffee grounds, 36
cleansing tools, 32
clove essential oil, 41, 156–157, 164
cocoa butter, 43–44, 113, 119, 162, 165
cocoa powder, 36, 59, 87, 123
coconut, 36
coconut butter, 44, 55, 76, 98, 100, 112, 118–119, 122, 127, 133, 136, 147, 151, 155, 157, 160, 162, 165
coconut flour, 55, 162
coconut milk, 36, 41, 50, 55, 83, 88, 100, 112, 118, 122, 127, 133, 142, 162–163
coconut oil, 41, 100, 118, 134, 143, 145
coconut sugar, 44, 87, 98, 112, 162
    replacing lacuma powder, 37
coconut yogurt, 133
coffee, 20, 28, 36, 80
coffee grinder, 29–30
coffee grounds, 23, 99, 111
combination skin, 16
    sample weekly regimen, 174
comfrey leaf, 93

comfrey leaf oil, 41
conditioners
    over the counter, 133
    pump or squeeze bottles, 31
cosmetics, toxicity of, 6–7
cotton or silk washcloths, 31
cotton rounds, 62
cranberry, 36
Crock-Pot, 31
cucumber, 36, 64, 66–67, 71

D

daily damage to skin
    bacteria, 19
    chemicals in skin-care products, 17
    harsh exfoliants, 18
    poor nutrition, 17–18
    stress, 19–20
    sun exposure, 18–19
Dalí, Salvador, 9
dandelion root, 36, 97
date sugar, 44, 87, 99
Dead Sea mud, 43, 80–81
Dead Sea salts, 168
decorative bottles and jars, 30–31
deep-pore masks, 22
dermatitis and cucumber, 36
dishrags, 32
distilled water, 48, 56, 59–60, 63–67, 70–72, 80, 84, 88–90, 94, 126, 158
double boiler, 30
Dr. Bonner's products, 127
dried alfalfa, 96
dried apricots, 90
dried birch, 96
dried cranberry, 90
dried herbs, 126
dried horsetail, 126
dried lavender petals, 126
dried mango, 90
dried nettle, 126
dried persimmon, 96

dried pineapple, 90
dried rosemary, 126
dry skin, 14–15
    bath vinegars, 109
    sample weekly regimen, 173
    solutions, 166

E

eczema and chamomile tea, 35
eggs, 45–46, 142, 145
egg whites, 85, 87, 132, 141
egg yolks, 134, 141
85/15 percent rule, 18
elderberries, 36, 91
elderflower, 36, 93
epidermis, 14
Epsom salt, 44, 107, 164, 168
essential oils, 20
    bath bomb, 25
    cautions, 41
exfoliants, 18
    almond meal, 33
    chia seeds, 35
    shredded coconut, 36
eyes, 28, 36

F

facial cleansers and almond milk, 33
facial steams, 22
    cooling off, 89
    immediately using, 91
fast food, 18
fenugreek, 36–37, 138
fixatives, 38
flavonoids, 35–37, 39
flavoring, 154
floral water. See hydrosols
French green clay, 43, 52, 60, 80
funnels, 29, 30

G

ginger, 37, 92, 99
ginseng, 37, 95

ACKNOWLEDGMENTS

The making of a book always involves more than you expect. Inevitably the undertaking includes many who never signed on for the task. Their support, input, and encouragement are key to the process and success.

My staff at *Sum*body was a huge advantage. I would call formulas into the lab and pick them up, modify them, take over the entire production for days in the lab with everyone mixing up and trying patches of products. Jenee, who not only runs the company, spent countless hours crunching numbers under crazy deadlines.

Thank you to all the willing and wonderful *Sum*body fans who bathed, made, washed, scrubbed, and combed all the products for review! Your thoughts and feedback were invaluable.

This was not an easy book to deliver! Throughout the entire (sometimes frustrating) process, my editor Nana proved to be a valuable asset.

The support and encouragement from my friends has been an invaluable pillar for me, with everything from proofreading to my dear friend Anne who came to the lab and made products as we were testing the ease of making them for beginners.

Diving back into work beyond caring for my father with dementia was not easy. A huge thank-you to his supportive staff, my husband, and my daughter who tried their best to pick up the slack, to keep him safe, happy, and entertained, and made this time possible.

I think it always goes without saying that not only is my family part of everything I do, but also without them none of this would be possible. My two daughters who have grown to be such amazing women are endless in their love and help. And of course Allen, who keeps making sure I understand the definition of pithy and never stops amusing me.

ABOUT THE AUTHOR

DEBORAH BURNES represents the new face of green living—modern, multifaceted, and holistic. As the CEO and co-founder of *Sum*body, a skin-care company dedicated to all-natural, eco-friendly products, Deborah has been profiled in *Luxury Spa Finder* magazine, which lauds her as being "at the forefront of the natural-beauty product revolution," and for her "commitment to purity" and "responsibly cultivated 'clean' ingredients."

A Native New Yorker, Deborah brings a unique blend of business savvy and approachable warmth to her interactions with everyday consumers, high-powered executives, and celebrities, and is considered one of the leading experts on natural skin care. Deborah has been a keynote speaker at industry events such as the Society of Cosmetic Chemists, HBA Global. Featured on television shows (such as the *Tyra Banks Show*, *Access Hollywood*, NBC's *Wine Country Living*, and *Lisa Oz Show*), in magazines (including *In Style*, *Lucky*, *Organic Style*, *Cosmopolitan*, *New Beauty*, *W*, *Shop Etc.*, and *O, The Oprah Magazine*), and in national newspapers and celebrity events like the Academy Awards, MTV Awards, and the Primetime Emmy Awards.

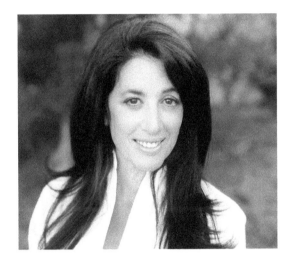

Deborah and *Sum*body have amassed thousands of devoted fans. Deborah combines knowledge of chemistry and biology with a background in cosmetology, natural medicine, and environmentalism, plus experience as a model, working mother, and beauty-industry insider. She synthesizes a vast amount of knowledge and experience from both the eco-sensitive and conventional sides of the fence, making her not only someone consumers can trust, but with whom they can identify with.